Modern Approach to Diagnosis and Treatment of Bladder Cancer

Edited by Francesco Ziglioli and Umberto Maestroni

Published in London, United Kingdom

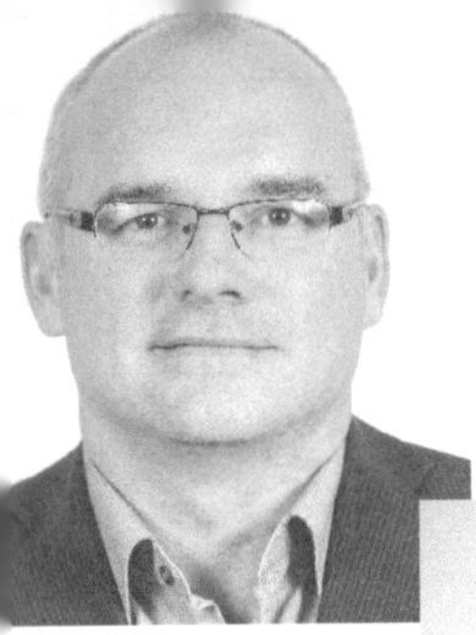
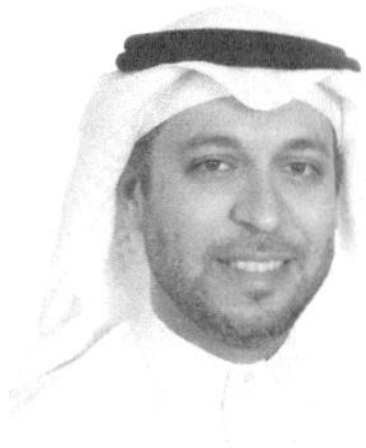
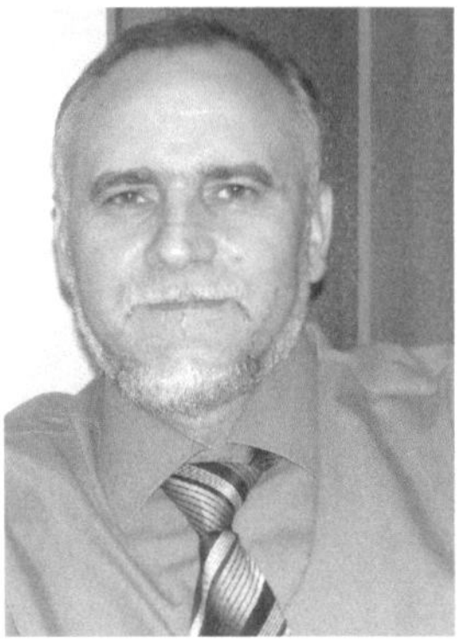
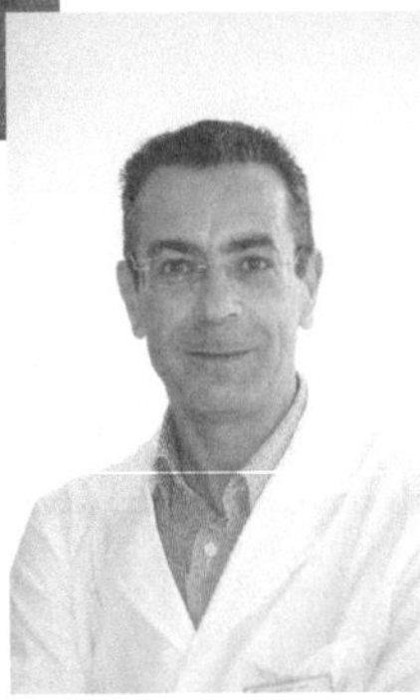
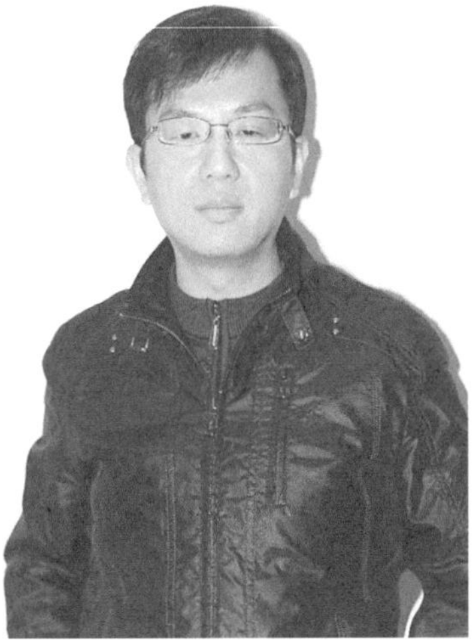
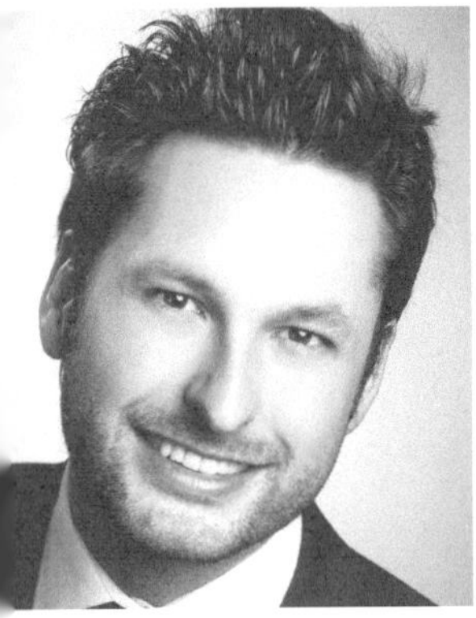
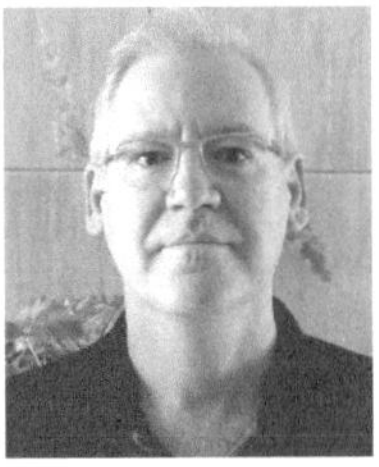

IntechOpen

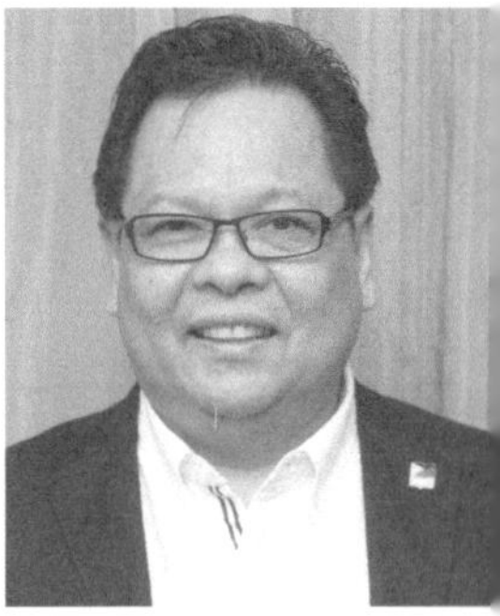
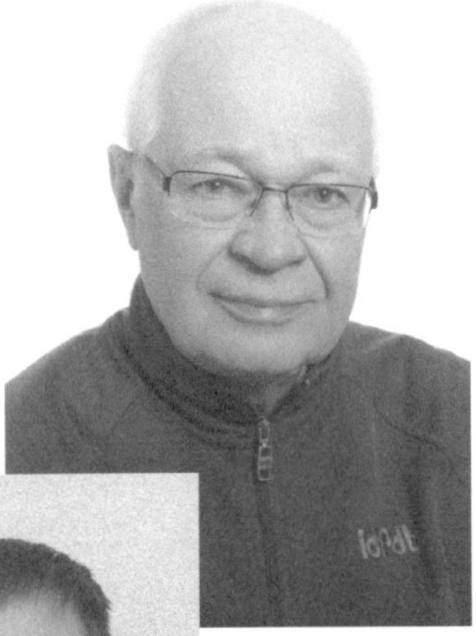
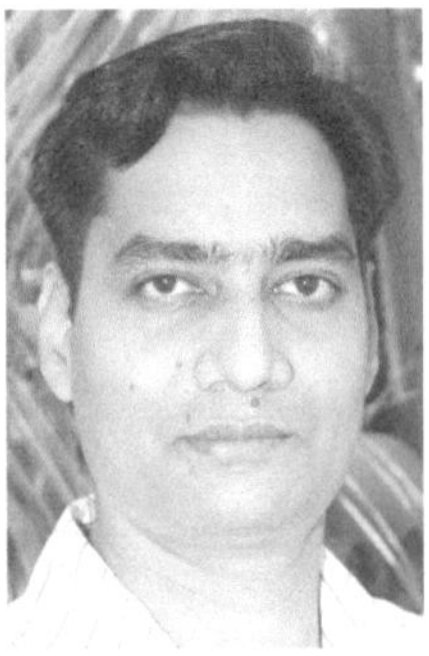
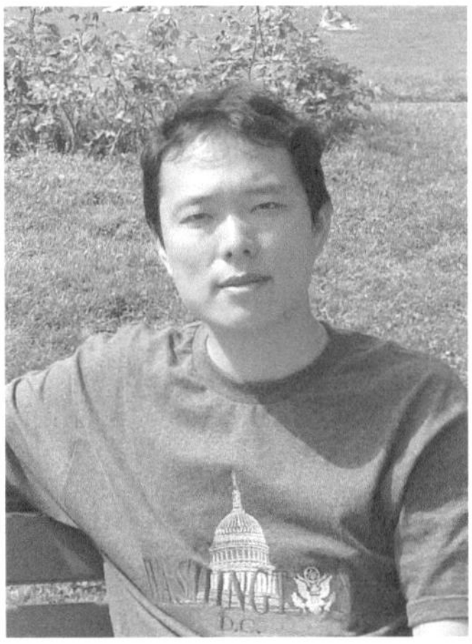
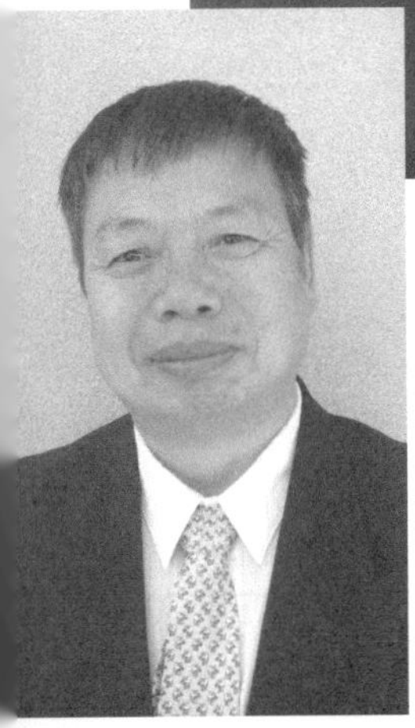
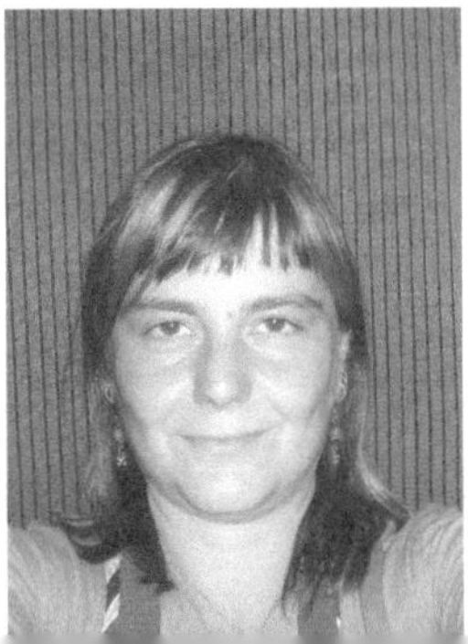

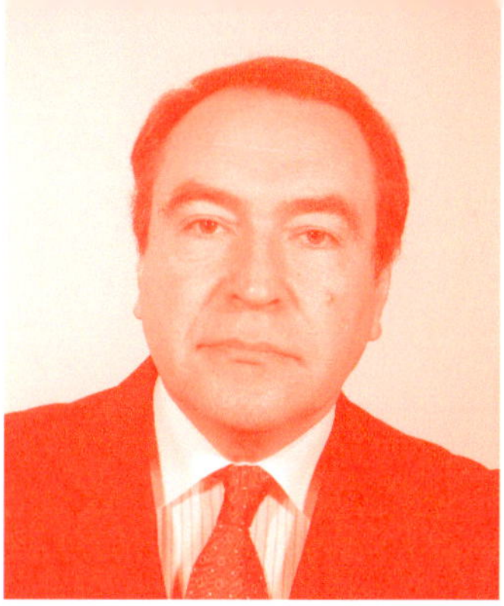

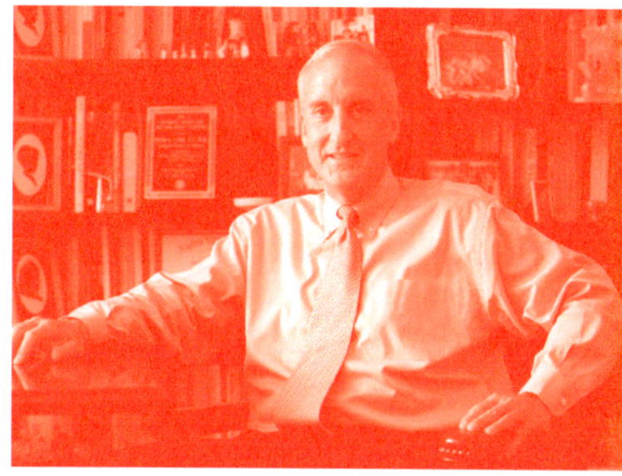

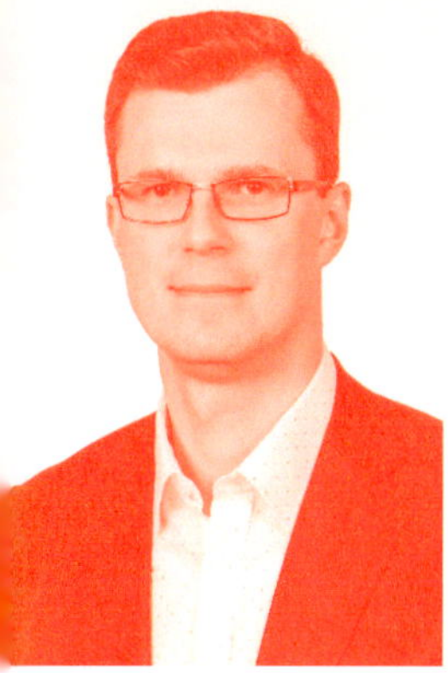

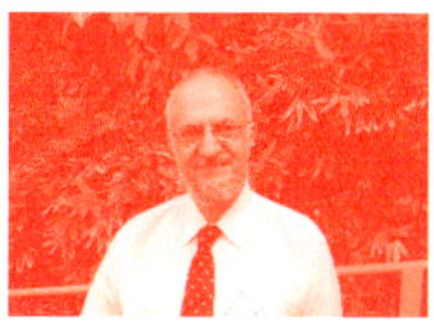

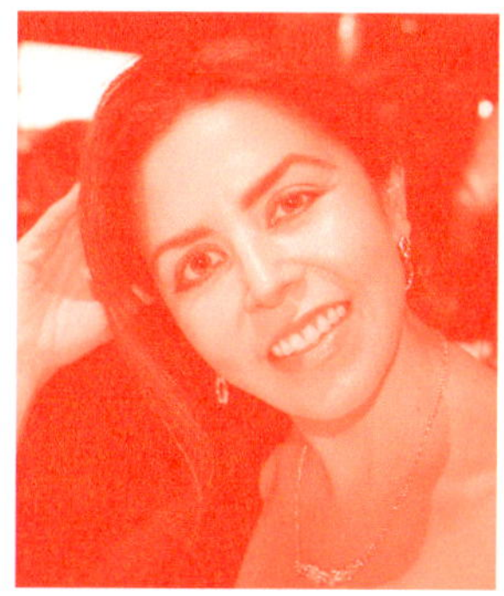

Supporting open minds since 2005

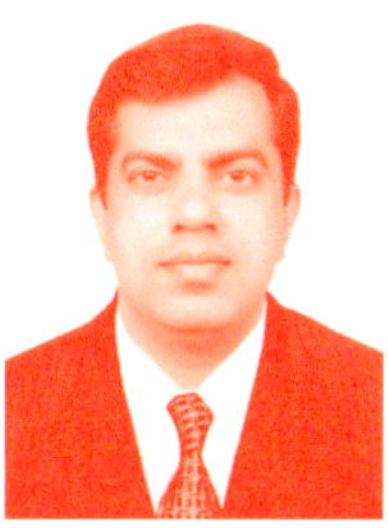

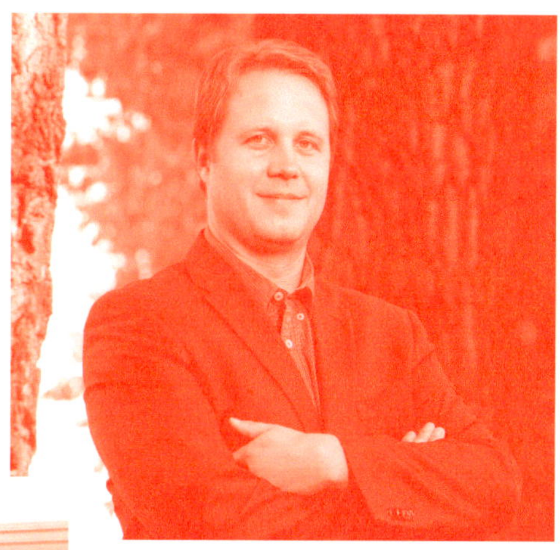

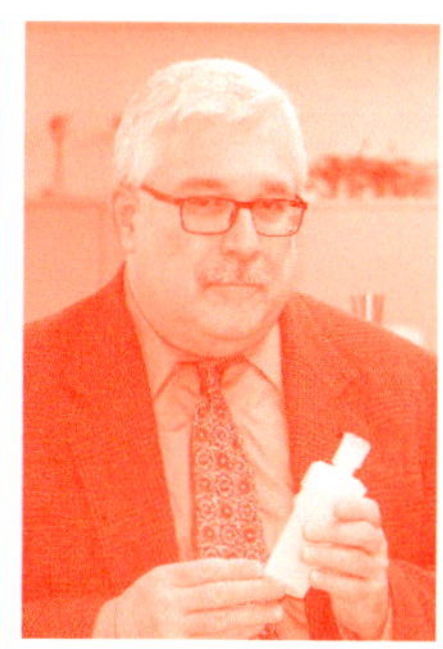

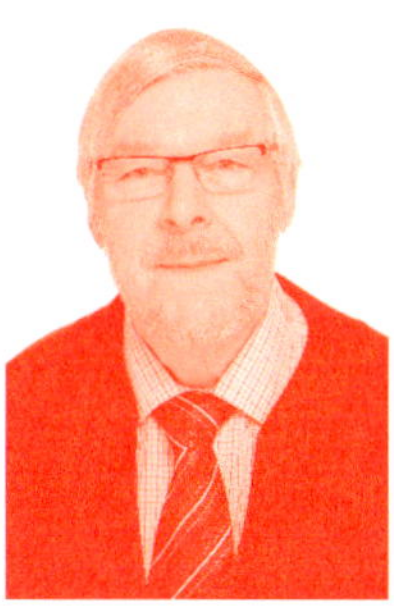

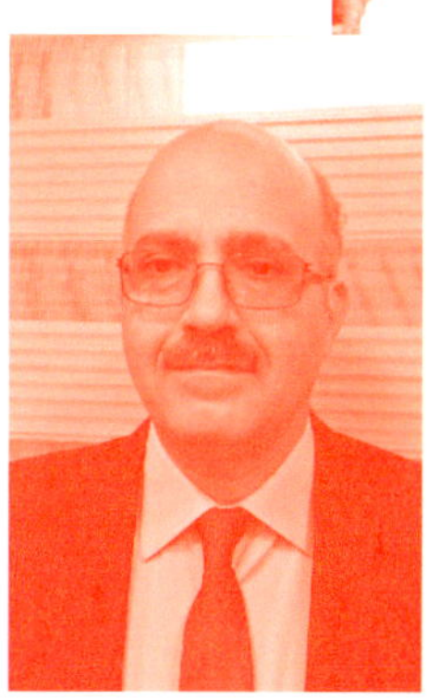

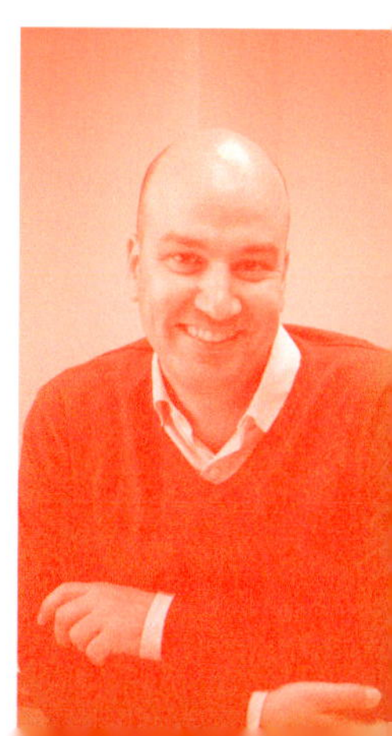

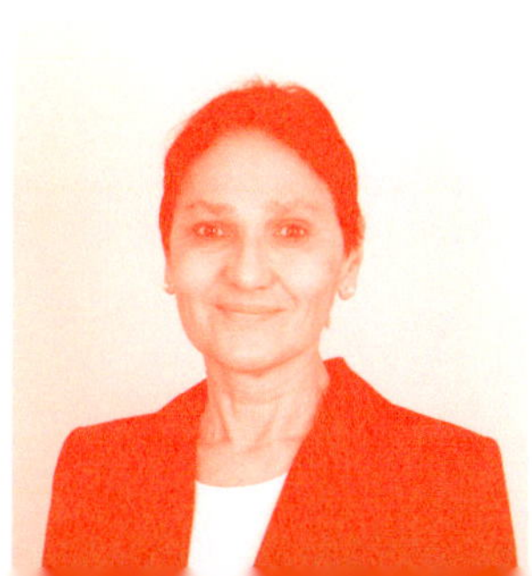

Modern Approach to Diagnosis and Treatment of Bladder Cancer
http://dx.doi.org/10.5772/intechopen.91525
Edited by Francesco Ziglioli and Umberto Maestroni

Contributors
Seema Kaushal, Hena Khandakar, Xue Li, Yingsheng Zhang, Dan Theodorescu, Pedro Ramos, Pedro Pereira, Paulo Dinis, Luís Pacheco-Figueiredo, Victor Enrique Corona-Montes, Eduardo Gonzalez-Cuenca, Richard Gaston, Juan Eduardo Sánchez-Núñez, Laurent López, Nikolaos Pardalidis, Panagiotis Pardalidis, Nikolaos Andriopoulos, Ankur Mittal, Vikas Kumar Panwar, Gurpremjit Singh

First published in London, United Kingdom, 2021 by IntechOpen
IntechOpen is the global imprint of INTECHOPEN LIMITED, registered in England and Wales, registration number: 11086078, 5 Princes Gate Court, London, SW7 2QJ, United Kingdom
Printed in Croatia

British Library Cataloguing-in-Publication Data
A catalogue record for this book is available from the British Library

Additional hard and PDF copies can be obtained from orders@intechopen.com

Modern Approach to Diagnosis and Treatment of Bladder Cancer
Edited by Francesco Ziglioli and Umberto Maestroni
p. cm.
Print ISBN 978-1-83969-190-4
Online ISBN 978-1-83969-191-1
eBook (PDF) ISBN 978-1-83969-192-8

Meet the editors

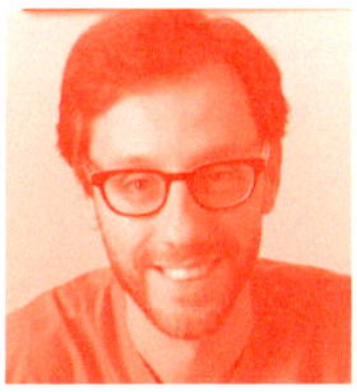

Francesco Ziglioli graduated from the University of Pavia, Italy, in 2006, and completed his residency in urology at the University Hospital of Parma, Italy, in 2012. After experience as a urologist in the United Kingdom, Dr. Ziglioli attended a fellowship in laparoscopy and robotic surgery at the Saint-Augustin Clinic, Bordeaux, France, in 2016. He currently works as a urologist at the Department of Urology, University Hospital of Parma. He is a fellow of the European Board of Urology and an editorial board member of three international journals. Dr. Ziglioli has published mainly in the field of prostate and kidney cancer.

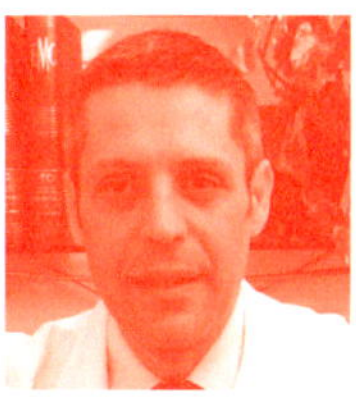

Umberto Maestroni graduated from the University of Bologna, Italy, in 1996, and completed his residency in general surgery at the University of Ferrara, Italy, in 2001, and in urology at the University of Parma, Italy, in 2007. He has been a rotating resident at the Department of Surgery, Division of Endoscopic Surgery, Cedars-Sinai Medical Center, Los Angeles, California, since 1999. He is the director of the Department of Urology, University Hospital of Parma, Italy. He is an editorial board member of three international journals and has published mainly in the fields of prostate cancer and other urologic diseases and treatments.

Contents

Preface

Bladder cancer is one of the most common carcinomas in urology. Advances in the diagnosis and treatment of this disease have led to important improvements in the oncologic and functional outcomes of patients, which are directly related to proper knowledge of the disease.

On one hand, conservative treatment strategies aim to preserve the bladder. On the other hand, robotic surgery can reduce the impact of adverse effects in those cases in which conservative treatment is not recommended.

The book begins with a review of bladder cancer, including molecular subtypes, the knowledge of which is key to understanding the behavior of different types of bladder cancer. Subsequent chapters discuss chemotherapy, immunotherapy, and minimally invasive techniques for surgical treatment.

Many experts have made this book a reality. Its completion would not have been possible without the efforts of many contributors. It is a pleasure for me to thank them all.

I would also like to acknowledge Maja and Ana for their precious support.

Francesco Ziglioli and Umberto Maestroni
University Hospital of Parma,
Italy

Chapter 1

Molecular Classification of Bladder Cancer

Seema Kaushal and Hena Khandakar

Abstract

Bladder cancer is a biologically and clinically heterogeneous disease. Traditional classification systems, based on pathologic grade, stage and clinical prognosis fail to fully explain how tumors with similar pathology exhibit diverse biological behavior. The introduction of transcriptomics technology has allowed us to catalog all of the mRNA expression patterns and DNA alterations in a given tumor thus expanding our understanding of human cancers. Molecular subtype profiling was attempted only recently in bladder cancer, with the earliest attempts dating back to 2010. Several different molecular classification systems have emerged since. Some of these systems address early bladder cancer, while others focus exclusively on the life-threatening muscle invasive tumors. These molecular subtypes have distinct morphological and clinical characteristics with different therapeutic and prognostic implications, particularly in the era of targeted therapies and immunotherapy. However, molecular subtyping is not without its limitations. Despite the rapidly expanding evidence for important clinical implications, much work is still needed to establish the utility (or lack thereof) of molecular subtyping, and its application in daily practice.

Keywords: molecular classification, muscle invasive bladder cancer, taxonomy, transcriptomics, targeted therapy

1. Introduction

Bladder cancer is the most common malignant tumor involving the urinary tract. Histologically, bladder cancers can be urothelial carcinomas, squamous cell carcinomas and adenocarcinomas, out of which urothelial carcinomas constitute over 90% [1]. Urothelial carcinoma is derived from the specialized epithelia of the bladder wall. Using a well-established differentiation program, basal stem cells at the stromal interface self-renew and generate intermediate and superficial urothelial cells to maintain and regenerate the urothelium in response to daily wear and tear. Bladder cancer results from the deregulation of this program. Conventionally, bladder cancer can be divided into non-muscle invasive bladder cancer (NMIBCs) and muscle invasive bladder cancers (MIBCs), based on the invasion of the muscularis propria. The low grade superficial NMIBCs and high grade MIBCs (HG MIBCs) develop along divergent molecular pathways of tumorigenesis and also show diverse biological behavior and molecular profile. Low grade NMIBCs constitute the majority of newly diagnosed bladder cancer cases, typically have a long protracted clinical course characterized by multiple recurrences, and require life-long monitoring, significantly contributing to bladder cancer morbidity. On the other hand, a large proportion of the MIBCs eventually metastasize, contributing to the bulk of bladder cancer mortality [2, 3].

Low grade papillary urothelial carcinomas occur due to fibroblast growth factor receptor 3 (FGFR3)/RAS/RAF pathway alterations, while the HG MIBCs develop along the TP53/RB1 mutation pathway [4, 5]. Chromosome 9 deletion occurs in the early phase of bladder cancer tumorigenesis. FGFR3/HRAS mutations frequently occur during the development of hyperplasia and low grade (Ta) carcinoma. Hyperplasia develops into high grade urothelial carcinoma (Ta) through the acquisition of CDKN2A alterations, which may progress to become T1 carcinoma after additional TP53/RB1 inactivation. TP53 mutations frequently occur during the development of urothelial dysplasia. These may develop into carcinoma in situ (Tis) after RB1 inactivation, which then progresses through non-muscle invasive infiltrating urothelial carcinomas (T1) to muscle invasive (T2) carcinoma.

Traditional classifications for bladder cancer are mainly based on pathological features and tumor stage. However, even with similar pathological staging and grading, recurrence and progression of bladder cancer shows marked heterogeneity, and directly affects optimal monitoring and treatment response. Only a proportion of cases of bladder cancer of a given grade and stage will progress to a higher stage. Thus the same treatment, such as, transurethral resection alone, or the administration of BCG or neoadjuvant chemotherapy may not be adequate for others. Some tumors are less likely to metastasise and need only local resection, while others are highly invasive and need radical cystectomy and/or other treatments. Currently, there is still no effective means to distinguish between the two. The pathological features of the tumor cannot fully reflect the "intrinsic characteristics" of bladder cancer.

With the rapid development of sequencing, mass spectrometry and other techniques, studies based on the '-omics' technology has transformed our understanding of human cancers. The basic method involves cataloging the entire mRNA expression pattern and DNA alteration profile by sequencing, microarray and other technologies and then performing a cluster analysis of the different genes based on gene expression levels and genes involved in a given biological process. After performing hierarchical cluster analysis on mRNA expression profiling data, clusters were validated by DNA PCR and/or immunohistochemistry (IHC), DNA methylation profiling, miRNA or lncRNA analysis. Among the earliest applications of this approach was to define intrinsic molecular subtypes in human breast cancer by Perou et al., [6]. Subsequently, over the last decade, molecular subtypes with distinct clinical behavior, histology and response to treatment were identified in other malignancies e.g. colon cancer, gliomas, acute leukemias and so on. Molecular subtype profiling was applied only recently in bladder cancer, with the earliest attempts dating back to 2010. Several different molecular classification systems have emerged since, with four standing out in the MIBCs, developed by Lund University group [7–10], The Cancer Genome Atlas (TCGA) consortium [11, 12], MD Anderson Cancer Centre [13] and the University of North Carolina [14]. Several other studies have followed up, in an attempt to unify [15] and reach a consensus [16] between the classification systems. Although each group defended the existence of a different numbers of subtypes (n = 2–6), there was remarkable overall concordance among the groups (**Table 1**). At the highest level, all classification systems recognized the existence of intrinsic luminal and non-luminal (basal) subtypes, which resembled normal luminal/intermediate and basal urothelial cells in gene expression profile.

For the two major types of bladder cancer, NMIBC and MIBC, molecular subtyping of bladder cancer can be divided into early subtyping (which included both NMIBC and MIBC), NMIBC subtyping and MIBC subtyping (**Table 2**).

TCGA [12]	Lund [8]	MDACC [13]	UNC [14]	Properties
Cluster I	UroA, GU	Luminal	Luminal	FGFR mutations, papillary histology
Cluster II	Infiltrated	p53-like	Luminal	CAFs, immune cells
Cluster III	SCC-like, UroB	Basal	Basal	Stem cell markers, squamous differentiation
Cluster IV	Infiltrated	p53-like	Claudin-low	EMTs, CAFs, immune cells

Table 1.
Table showing overlap between the subtypes in the initial classification systems and the cardinal properties of these subtypes, adapted from McConkey et al. [17], CAF-cancer associated fibroblasts, EMT- epithelial-mesenchymal transition.

Subtyping systems	Abbreviation	Number of cases	Subtypes
Early BC subtyping system	Lund 2012 [8] 5 subtypes	n = 308	Urobasal A, genomically unstable, infiltrated, urobasal B and squamous cell carcinoma-like
	Baylor tumor differentiation classification 2012 [19] 3 subtypes	n = 492	Basal, intermediate, and differentiated
NMIBC subtyping	UROMOL 2016 [20] 3 subtypes	n = 400	Class1, 2 and 3
	Van Kessel 2018 [21] 3 subtypes	n = 1239	EAU high risk NMIBCs classified into good, moderate and poor prognostic subtypes
MIBC subtyping	UNC 2014 [14] 2 subtypes	n = 262	Basal-like (including claudin-low), and luminal
	MDACC 2014 [13] 2 subtypes	n = 83	Luminal, p53-like and basal
	TCGA 2014 [12] 4 subtypes	n = 129	Clusters I, II, III and IV
	TCGA 2017 [11] 5 subtypes	n = 412	Luminal-papillary, luminal (not-specified), luminal-infiltrated, basal-squamous, neural
	Consensus classification 2019 [16] 6 subtypes	n = 1750	Luminal-papillary, luminal not specified, luminal unstable, stroma-rich, basal/squamous, and neuroendocrine-like
BC subtyping with both NMIBCs and MIBCs	BOLD 2018 [22] 6 subtypes	n = 2411	Neural-like, luminal-like, papillary-like, HER2-like, squamous cell carcinoma-like and mesenchymal-like

Table 2.
Summary of major molecular subtyping systems, adapted from Zhu et al., 2020 [18].

2. Early bladder cancer subtyping systems

The earliest representative studies on the molecular classification of bladder cancer were conducted by Sjödahl et al. at the University of Lund, initially proposed in 2010 and finalized in 2012 and the tumor differentiation classification by Chan et al., of the Baylor University group, 2012 [19]. The Baylor classification focused on tumor biology. They proposed a KRT14/Thy-1/CD44 expressing cancer stem cells as the bladder cancer precursor. This cancer stem cell evolved into a partially differentiated KRT5/KRT17/CD44-positive progeny, which in turn acquired KRT8/18 expression and eventually differentiated into luminal cells expressing uroplakins and KRT20. Tumors were classified into basal, intermediate and differentiated classes based on their resemblance to normal urothelial differentiation. Based on the above classification, the KRT14 group (basal subtype) showed the poorest prognosis and were also found to be resistant to neoadjuvant cisplatin-based chemotherapy.

The Lund University group initially defined two intrinsic molecular subtypes named as MS1 and MS2 based on gene expression, genomic, and gene mutation levels by whole genome comparative genomic hybridization and mutation studies [7]. By combining molecular and pathologic data, it was possible to divide tumors into grade 1 or 2 (MS1) and grade 3 (MS2) (WHO1999), and into Ta (MS1) and $\geq$ T2 (MS2) stages based on the MS1 and MS2 subtypes.

Subsequently, an extensive biological interpretation of gene expression data identified that biological themes including immune, late cell cycle, keratin, receptor tyrosine kinases and FGFR3 signatures determined their data structure. Based on tumor histopathology, gene signatures, and status of FGFR3, PIK3CA, and TP53 mutations, three major subtypes of UC were defined: urobasal (Uro) (further subdivided into MS1a, MS1b, and MS2b2.1), genomically unstable (GU) (MS2a1 and MS2a2), and SCC-like (SCCL) (MS2b2.2) [8]. Subsequent studies also identified an "infiltrated" group in which the stromal inflammatory transcripts were prominently expressed. Among the urobasal tumors (MS2b2.1), a subset showed "progressed phenotype" with aberrant expression of basal keratins in suprabasal cell layers and upregulation of late cell cycle activity. These tumors were mostly large and invasive, and were named urobasal B to distinguish it from urobasal A tumors that were non-muscle invasive in almost all cases. The molecular subtypes thus defined, transcended pathological staging and all four subtypes (UroA, UroB, GU, and SCCL) were detected among T1 tumors. The initial Lund taxonomic studies included both NMIBC and MIBC and subsequent studies focussed predominantly on MIBC classification.

3. Molecular subtyping of early-stage bladder cancer

Variability in terminology has created a challenge in the molecular classification of early-stage bladder cancer. Treating clinicians emphasize the dichotomous division of BCs into NMIBC and MIBC, and often lump all NMIBCs together when planning molecular studies. In contrast pathologists tend to see a stark difference between non-invasive tumors and invasive tumors limited to the lamina propria and classify accordingly.

Molecular diversity in non-invasive BC differs from that of MIBC. Non-invasive BC histologically includes papillary UC and flat CIS, although both may co-exist in the same patient. As we have discussed earlier, low-grade non-invasive papillary UC has a high frequency of FGFR3 mutation. LGUC progresses to HGUC and invasive carcinoma through the acquisition of TP53 mutations and 9p21 loss involving the gene encoding CDKN2A. In contrast, most CIS lesions have TP53 mutations early in evolution and do not acquire FGFR3 mutations [4, 5].

In the Lund system [8], majority of non-invasive UCs are urothelial-like, while CIS may be either urothelial-like or genomically unstable. They identified a "CIS signature" by utilizing a 16-gene classifier which was specifically expressed in flat

CIS, as well as in early-stage invasive carcinoma with associated CIS, and a large proportion of MIBCs of the basal-squamous subtype. In addition, MIBCs with concurrent CIS had greater genomic instability compared with those without it. Although majority of non-invasive papillary UCs were of luminal subtype, there is substantial molecular diversity among cases. The most clinically relevant diversity was related to cell cycle regulatory genes. Tumors with greater activation of the cell cycle had higher rates of recurrence and progression to MIBCs.

The UROMOL study of 2016 [20] evaluated expression profiles of NMIBCs including non-invasive papillary UC and invasive UC limited to the lamina propria (stage T1). A few cases of CIS and a small group of MIBCs were also included for comparison. Tumors were classified into 3 subtypes based on relative expression of luminal and basal-squamous markers and cell cycle activity. Three subtypes were proposed, named as Type 1 (early cell cycle activation and higher luminal gene expression), Type 3 (early cell cycle activation with lower luminal gene expression) and Type 2 (late cell cycle activation). Type 2 tumors, which included the highest proportion of T1 samples, had the greatest propensity to progress to muscle invasion. On the other hand, expression of luminal genes did not significantly affect patient outcome. In addition, non-invasive papillary tumors also varied in the degree of chromosomal instability. The unstable group had tumors with higher proliferation, greater mutational burden, and high-grade histology.

Von Kessel et al., in 2018 [21], determined that methylation status of GATA2, TBX2, TBX3 and ZIC4 and mutations in FGFR3, TERT, PIK3CA, and RAS correlated with progression rates of NMIBC. Wild-type FGFR3 and GATA2 and TBX3 methylation were significantly correlated with NMIBC progression. Thus, high risk NMIBC group was reclassified into good, moderate and poor prognostic classes with low, medium and high risk of progression.

However, because molecular subtyping of non–muscle-invasive bladder cancer has not demonstrated clear value in clinical decision making, it is not currently recommended to incorporate it on a routine basis, as per the ISUP recommendations published in 2020.

4. Molecular subtyping of MIBC

Much of the work on molecular subtyping of bladder cancer has been undertaken with MIBCs in consideration and an increasing number of classification systems have emerged with four of them standing out (**Figure 1**). Although the subtypes within these systems are largely similar, they differ in clinically and biologically meaningful ways.

The UNC classification proposed by Damrauer et al. [14], used K2 consensus clustering, to divide tumors into basal (KRT5/6 and CD44) vs. luminal (PPARG, GATA3, KRT20, and UPK2) subtypes utilizing a 47 gene classifier, BASE47. The basal subtype showed similarities with the basal subtype of breast cancers, as demonstrated by applying the PAM50 signature to their dataset. In addition, like in breast cancers, a claudin-low subgroup was identified among basal tumors. The claudin-low subgroup had outcomes similar to basal tumors and was rich in epithelial-mesenchymal transition (EMT) signatures and tumor initiating cell markers. A significant enrichment in genes related to inflammatory cell infiltration and immune checkpoint was also seen in the basal subgroup and, more specifically, among the claudin-low tumors. There was no significant difference in TP53 pathway alterations in the subtypes. The basal subtype, which was more frequent among females, had a high rate of RB pathway gene alterations, while the luminal subtype was rich in FGFR3 and TSC1mutations.

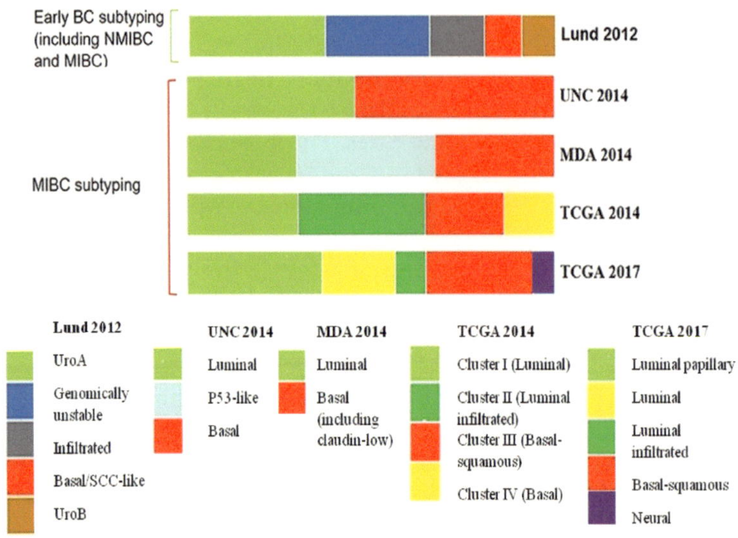

Figure 1.
Figure showing the similarities between the molecular subtypes in the different classification systems. Luminal and basal subtypes exist in all classification systems (figure adapted from Zhu et al. [18]).

The MDA group [13] also classified BC into basal, p53-like and luminal tumors similar to breast cancer. Their luminal and p53-like subtypes had similar mRNA profiles but wild-type p53 gene was significantly activated in the p53-like subtype. All three subtypes had similar frequency of p53 mutations, but the p53-ness contributed by increased wild-type p53 expression was thought to contribute to chemo-resistance in the p53-subtype. The basal subtype was enriched in squamous cell differentiation markers and activated p63 and was more invasive with poorer clinical prognosis.

The TCGA 2014 [12] subtyped MIBCs into four clusters numbered I to IV utilizing an integrated genomic analysis of chemotherapy-naive, invasive UCs by analyzing for somatic mutations, DNA copy number alterations, mRNA and microRNA expression profile, as well as protein analysis, and DNA methylation studies. Cluster I predominantly exhibited papilloma phenotype and was enriched in FGFR3 mutations. Both cluster I and II expressed GATA3, FOXA1, UPK3A transcription factors and uroplakin family of genes and were enriched in RBB2 mutations and ER beta. Cluster III expressed squamoid phenotype and its associated keratin expression. Subsequently in 2017, TCGA expanded their classification [11] into five distinct subtypes, diving luminal tumors into three subtypes, luminal papillary, luminal and luminal infiltrated. They also included a neural subtype in addition to the earlier described basal subtype.

4.1 Intrinsic molecular subtypes and intra-tumor heterogeneity

Intrinsic molecular subtype, a term which first used in breast carcinomas [6] refers to subtypes which reflect an intrinsic property of the tumor. The luminal and basal intrinsic subtypes reflect the property of the tumor cells to show urothelial or basal stem-cell-like differentiation signatures [23].

However, transcriptomic studies identified the entire genetic signature of a tumor, which in the case of invasive malignancies, included variable components of stromal and immune signatures. Thus, in addition to the two intrinsic subtypes, some of the subtypes defined in the various study groups were based on the characteristics of the tumor-stroma or tumor infiltrating inflammatory cells such as the p53-like'subtype [13], infiltrated subtype [8], luminal-infiltrated subtype [11] as examples. These non-intrinsic subtypes could be recognized as a property of the stroma or inflammatory cells when studies were performed later which localized the gene expression patterns in situ, by immunohistochemistry [10, 23, 24]. Many of these non-intrinsic subtypes could be resolved into luminal and basal subtypes based on tumor phenotype on immunohistochemistry, while others continued to express non-luminal, non-basal phenotype, like the double negative subtype of Dadhania et al., [24].

4.1.1 Intrinsic luminal subtype

At the top of the hierarchical level, MIBCs were divided into luminal-like and nonluminal-like classes based on the presence or absence of bimodally expressed urothelial differentiation signature.

About half of the MIBCs expressed this signature characterized by the expression of KRT20, UPK1–3 (uroplakin 1, 2 and 3), epithelial biomarkers (E-cadherin/CDH1 and members of the miR-200 family), along with transcriptional regulators PPARG (peroxisome proliferator activated receptor-γ), GRHL2–3 (grainyhead like transcription factor), ELF3 and TBX2–3. Luminal MIBCs also displayed active Estrogen Receptor/TRIM24 pathway gene expression and were enriched with FOXA1, GATA3, ERBB2 and ERBB3 expressed on superficial (umbrella cells) and intermediate cells of the normal urothelium [7]. There was increased expression of fibroblast growth factor receptor-3 (FGFR3), with activating FGFR3 mutations in the most differentiated luminal tumors.

The luminal tumors were further sub-stratified into urothelial-like (UroA, UroB and UroC) and genomically unstable (GU) subtypes by the Lund University group [8], luminal papillary, luminal and luminal infiltrated subtypes by TCGA [11] and luminal papillary, luminal non-specified, and luminal unstable subtypes in the Consensus classification [16].

The urothelial-like tumors expressed FGFR3 and CCND1, and frequently showed 9p21 (CDKN2A) loss. On immunohistochemistry, only the urothelial-like tumors retained the basal stratification seen in normal urothelium and express CK5 at least focally, particularly at the tumor-stroma interface [9, 10]. Similar to UroA tumors in the Lund classification, the luminal-papillary subtype in TCGA and Consensus classification were also characterized by FGFR3 mutations; by papillary histology; and by low carcinoma-in-situ scores. Such cancers had a low risk for progression, and while preliminary data suggests a low likelihood of response to cisplatin-based NACT [25], they may respond to tyrosine kinase inhibitors of FGFR3 family [26, 27] or to PPARγ-inhibitors [10] or to Estrogen receptor modulators [28].

Genomically unstable subtype (GU) of luminal tumors expressed FOXM1 and absent to low levels of FGFR3, but not KRT5 [9]. They also frequently showed RB1 loss, and had a high rate of TP53 mutations. Highest ERBB2 expression is also seen in GU subtype. Although they showed urothelial differentiation signature, GU tumors were in fact poorly differentiated and frequently high grade on histology [9, 10]. On immunohistochemistry, they did not express CK5, but expressed late cell cycle makers such as p16 [10]. The luminal unstable subtype of Consensus classification showed similar features to the GU subtype described by Lund University group. These tumors may respond to drugs targeting ERBB2 [23].

In terms of prognosis, luminal papillary tumors or UroA tumors had very good prognosis, while the GU subtype showed an intermediate prognosis compared to urothelial-like and basal/SCC-like tumors [10, 12, 16].

4.1.2 Intrinsic non-luminal subtype: Basal and neuronal

Intrinsic non-luminal MIBC included basal MIBC (Choi et al., 2014) [13] and neuronal or small cell neuroendocrine MIBC. The basal subtype has been renamed basal-squamous in the later classification systems as it is characterized by squamous differentiation [8, 12].

Basal-squamous MIBCs expressed signal biomarkers similar to normal basal cells in the urothelium like high molecular weight cytokeratins KRT1, KRT5, KRT6, KRT14, KRT16, 15 KRT6A, KRT6B, KRT6C and CD44 and CDH3 [8, 11]. However, unlike normal basal urothelial cells which retained urothelial differentiation factors (GATA3 and PPARG), the basal-squamous subtype showed down-regulation of this signature. Interestingly, they had a higher incidence in females unlike all the other subtypes which were male predominant [11].

Basal MIBCs were also characterized by up-regulation of the epidermal growth factor receptor (EGFR) and other ligands of the epidermal differentiation complex such as S100A7 and SPRR1B, similar to basal breast and head and neck squamous cell carcinomas. Cell cycle regulator p63 played a central role in controlling the basal pathway of differentiation, and STAT3, NFκB, and Hypoxia Induced Factor-1α (HIF-1α) were also involved [23].

Without treatment, basal MIBCs had poorer survival [13, 14] but they responded well to neoadjuvant chemotherapy [11]. Because NACT pathological complete response is associated with excellent long-term survival, aggressive early management of basal MIBCs with NACT offers the best chance for improved survival for these patients.

This subtype also had the strongest immune expression signature, including T cell markers, inflammation genes and lymphocytic infiltrates. It is predicted that the basal-squamous subtype may respond to anti-PD-L1, anti-PD-1 and anti-CTLA-4 agents [28, 29]. EGFR-, NFκB, HIF-1α/VEGF, and/or STAT3-targeted agents may also have a role within this subtype [27].

The neuronal subtype showed no histopathological distinction from other types of MIBC in most cases. Nonetheless, they had high levels of TP53 and RB1 mutations, similar to small cell carcinomas in other tissues. It had the worst survival of the mRNA expression subtypes, making it important to recognize [10, 11].

4.1.3 Non-intrinsic subtypes: P53-like, luminal-infiltrated, stromal-like, infiltrated, claudin-low

P53-like MIBCs showed some overlap in gene expression with luminal and basal subtypes of the UNC classification but were characterized by the expression of an active wild-type p53-associated gene expression signature [13]. P53-like subtype of bladder cancer responded poorly to neo-adjuvant chemotherapy [13, 28, 30]. Wild-type p53-induced reversible senescence and quiescence had been implicated in causing chemo-resistance. However, even though p53-associated expression signatures were present, *TP53* mutation frequencies were found to be similar in luminal, p53-like and basal subtypes defined by Choi et al., (2014). The p53-ness as measured by mRNA expression was found to be a more accurate predictor of de novo and induced MIBC chemo-resistance than analysis of *TP53* mutational status [23].

The luminal-infiltrated subtype reported by the TCGA was characterized by low tumor purity, with high expression of epithelial-mesenchymal transition (EMT) and myofibroblast markers, and of the miR-200 s. It showed medium expression of PD-L1 and CTLA4 immune markers. This subtype had been reported to respond to immune checkpoint inhibitors like Anti-PD-L1 [29].

Stromal-like subtype from the Consensus classification, the infiltrated subtype from the Lund classification [10] and claudin-low subtype of the MD Anderson Cancer Centre classification [14] all showed similar features of low-tumor purity, high EMT and stromal related transcripts with increased cancer stem cell-like gene expression profile. Claudin-low tumors described by Damrauer et al. [14], in addition, showed increased expression of claudins-1, 3, and 7 and had a similar expression profile to the claudin-low breast cancer subtype. Dadhania et al., [24] in their meta-analysis of the TCGA, Lund and MD Anderson cohorts also identified a subset of tumors with low urothelial and basal expression signatures, which they termed "double negative", which showed similar expression profile to claudin-low tumors.

With tumor progression, alterations are seen both in the intrinsic characteristics of the tumor cell, as well as in the tumor microenvironment (TME). Early MIBC molecular classification systems mainly focused on the molecular classification of tumor cells themselves. With a deeper understanding of BC cells and their TME, molecular subtyping efforts have begun to focus more on intratumor heterogeneity, stromal-extracellular matrix (ECM) interactions and immune cell infiltration, allowing further refinement of the molecular subtypes. Currently, studies on molecular subtyping are mainly based on whole tumor DNA or RNA studies rather than focusing on a single tumor cell. In this method, intratumoral heterogeneity can greatly affect the accuracy of molecular subtyping. Warrick et al. [31] conducted a pathological examination on 309 bladder cancer markers and found that nearly one fourth of them exhibited intratumoral variation in tissue samples. Out of the 83 specimens subtyped by them with the Lund subtyping system, 39% exhibited molecular heterogeneity. Even among the subtypes, the basal-squamous subtype particularly showed the greatest variability; with approximately 78% of these tumors simultaneously exhibiting the genomically unstable or urothelial-like subtype.

Several immunohistochemistry based algorithms have been developed in an attempt to classify bladder cancer into clinically and prognostically significant molecular subtypes [9, 10, 24, 32]. The use of immunohistochemistry as a surrogate to molecular testing shows promise in making molecular subtyping amenable to widespread use. The use of a simple panel comprising of a luminal urothelial markers like GATA3 and basal keratin marker like KRT5 can help identify a GATA3 positive, KRT5 low luminal subtype and a GATA3 negative, KRT5 high basal subtype. Tumors which are negative for GATA3 and have low keratin may be further tested for mesenchymal or neuroendocrine markers. The luminal tumors may also be further subtyped into uro-like tumors which are p16 negative and genomically unstable tumors which show p16 positivity [33]. The subtypes thus identified have demonstrated significant prognostic and predictive value [24, 32].

5. Clinical significance of molecular subtypes of bladder cancer

Not only do clinical outcomes differ among the molecular subtypes, but also therapeutic response. The gold-standard for management of MIBCs for disease confined to the pelvis includes radical cystectomy preceded by platinum based neo-adjuvant chemotherapy. Although a significant minority of patients treated this way achieves durable response and improved cancer specific survival, a sizeable fraction does not respond. In fact, a meta-analysis has suggested that there is only 5% absolute survival benefit at 5 years for patients treated in this manner [34]. In addition, concerns regarding delayed surgery and risk of serious morbidity have limited the usage rates of NACT for cystectomy patients at 25% or less [35, 36]. Biomarker tests that predict chemo-response could address these problems by identifying patients most likely to benefit. In this regard, data suggests that NAC confers the greatest benefit in basal tumors [11, 29], while the "p53-like subtype" has been reported to confer chemo-resistance [13]. However, current ISUP working group guidelines of 2020 do not recommend routine subtyping to guide NACT [37].

Data published by the TCGA Consortium stated that about 69% of BCs contain potentially actionable therapeutic targets which associate with specific molecular subtypes [11]. Mutations and amplifications of FGFR3 are seen in 50–80% of superficial bladder cancers and up to 20% of MIBCs [19]. Luminal-papillary tumors demonstrate a high rate of these alterations [11]; however, clinical trials have not yet incorporated molecular classification to determine patient eligibility. Similarly PIK3CA is also a frequently mutant gene and therapies targeting PI3K pathway have also shown preclinical BC trials [38]. Other targets such as ERBB2 and TSC1 are also being investigated as therapeutic targets.

Molecular subtyping may also provide a guide to BC immunotherapy. Anti-programmed death 1 (PD-1) and anti-programmed death-ligand 1(PD-L1) and cytotoxic T-lymphocyte antigen 4 (CTLA-4) are important second line therapies for MIBC with NAC failure. A few are also approved as first line therapy for cisplatin ineligible cases. Unfortunately, not all patients benefit from immunotherapy [39, 40]. Testing for biomarkers of response involves IHC for PD-1 or PD-L1 or estimation of tumor mutation burden, micro-satellite instability or immune-microenvironment of the tumor. However, none of these biomarkers have shown overwhelming predictive efficacy over others [41–43]. The luminal infiltrated subtype in the TCGA 2017 subtyping system was found to be enriched in PD-L1, CTLA-4 and other immune signatures. In particular, although this subtype did not respond well to NACT, they showed good response to anti-PD-L1 and anti-PD-1 treatment. The basal subtype has also shown response to immunotherapeutic agents in addition to being sensitive to NACT [11, 29]. Molecular subtypes may thus help define patient selection for immunotherapy.

6. Conclusion

Compared to traditional classification of BCs, molecular subtypes provide more information regarding tumor biology, prognosis and treatment. In general, BC can be divided into luminal and non-luminal subtypes based on their degree of urothelial differentiation. The luminal subtype is further subdivided into those with papillary features, which are superficial, predominantly non-invasive. Though they carry good prognosis when compared to other treatment-naïve subtypes, they do not respond well to conventional NAC and may benefit from targeted therapies. The luminal infiltrated type has more inflammatory and stromal signatures. They are more invasive than luminal papillary tumors and may respond well to immunotherapies. Basal/squamous tumors express stem cell and squamous differentiation associated gene expression signatures. They are aggressive untreated, but respond well to NACT as well as immunotherapies but are insensitive to radiotherapy. The neural subtype forms a minority of non-luminal tumors with neuronal or neuroendocrine phenotype and usually carry poor prognosis but respond to NACT. There are an increasing number of molecular subtyping systems being constantly updated. While they carry great potential to reform BC prognostication and therapeutics, they are not entirely without limitations. Accessibility is a key issue in the present times. Molecular subtyping is mainly based on "static" research, especially in NMIBC, and enables a one-time detection and analysis of tumor specimens rather than "dynamic" tracking to over the disease course. It has also mainly focused on genome and transcriptome research so far but proteomics and immune status of tumors are also closely related to their development. Therefore, the implementation of multiomics is a key necessity in future studies on molecular subtyping. Intratumor heterogeneity also provides another challenge with patient outcome being dominated by one subtype more than the other. With the rapid development of single-cell high-throughput sequencing, mass spectrometric analysis, immune cell analysis and other technologies, the accuracy of the molecular subtyping prediction system need further improvement. Compared to the existing classification system, molecular subtyping methods offer a more comprehensive analysis, particularly to guide adjuvant chemotherapy, targeted therapy and immunotherapy. In the future, these classifications will become an important complementary approach to traditional pathological classification.

Conflict of interest

The authors declare no conflict of interest.

Author details

Seema Kaushal* and Hena Khandakar
Department of Pathology, All India Institute of Medical Sciences, New Delhi, India

*Address all correspondence to: seema.dr@gmail.com

References

[1] Holger Moch, Peter A. Humphrey, Thomas M. Ulbright, Victor E. Reuter (Eds): WHO Classification of tumors of the Urinary System and Male Genital Organs (4th Edition) 2016, 86-93.

[2] Botteman MF, Pashos CL, Redaelli A, Laskin B, Hauser R. The health economics of bladder cancer: a comprehensive review of the published literature. PharmacoEconomics. 2003; 21:1315-1330. [PMID: 14750899]

[3] Shah JB, McConkey DJ, Dinney CP. New strategies in muscle-invasive bladder cancer: on the road to personalized medicine. Clinical cancer research: an official journal of the American Association for Cancer Research. 2011;17:2608-2612. [PMID: 21415213]

[4] Knowles, M.A.; Hurst, C.D. Molecular biology of bladder cancer: New insights into pathogenesis and clinical diversity. Nat. Rev. Cancer 2015, 15, 25-41.

[5] Wu, X.R. Urothelial tumourigenesis: A tale of divergent pathways. Nat. Rev. Cancer 2005, 5, 713-725.

[6] Perou CM, Sørlie T, Eisen MB, van de Rijn M, Jeffrey SS, Rees CA, et al. Molecular portraits of human breast tumors. Nature. 2000 Aug 1;406(6797):747-52. 1.

[7] Lindgren D, Frigyesi A, Gudjonsson S, Sjödahl G, Hallden C, Chebil G, et al. Combined Gene Expression and Genomic Profiling Define Two Intrinsic Molecular Subtypes of Urothelial Carcinoma and Gene Signatures for Molecular Grading and Outcome. Cancer Res. 2010 May 1;70(9):3463-3472.

[8] Sjödahl G, Lauss M, Lövgren K, Chebil G, Gudjonsson S, Veerla S, et al. A Molecular Taxonomy for Urothelial Carcinoma. Clin Cancer Res. 2012 Jun 15;18(12):3377-3386.

[9] Sjödahl G, Lövgren K, Lauss M, Patschan O, Gudjonsson S, Chebil G, et al. Toward a molecular pathologic classification of urothelial carcinoma. Am J Pathol. 2013 Sep;183(3):681-691.

[10] Sjödahl G, Eriksson P, Liedberg F, Höglund M. Molecular classification of urothelial carcinoma: global mRNA classification versus tumour-cell phenotype classification. J Pathol. 2017;242(1):113-125.

[11] Robertson AG, Kim J, Al-Ahmadie H, Bellmunt J, Guo G, Cherniack AD, et al. Comprehensive molecular characterization of muscle invasive bladder cancer. Cell. 2017 Oct 19;171(3):540-556.e25.

[12] Weinstein JN, Akbani R, Broom BM, Wang W, Verhaak RGW, McConkey D, et al. Comprehensive molecular characterization of urothelial bladder carcinoma. Nature. 2014 Mar;507(7492):315-322.

[13] Choi W, Porten S, Kim S, Willis D, Plimack ER, Hoffman-Censits J, et al. Identification of distinct basal and luminal subtypes of muscle-invasive bladder cancer with different sensitivities to frontline chemotherapy. Cancer Cell. 2014 Feb 10;25(2):152-165.

[14] Damrauer JS, Hoadley KA, Chism DD, Fan C, Tiganelli CJ, Wobker SE, et al. Intrinsic subtypes of high-grade bladder cancer reflect the hallmarks of breast cancer biology. Proc Natl Acad Sci USA. 2014 Feb 25;111(8):3110-5. 1.

[15] Aine M, Eriksson P, Liedberg F, Höglund M, Sjödahl G. On Molecular Classification of Bladder Cancer: Out of One, Many. European Urology. 2015 Dec 1;68(6):921-923.

[16] Kamoun A, Reyniès A de, Allory Y, Sjödahl G, Robertson AG, Seiler R, et al. A Consensus Molecular Classification of Muscle-invasive Bladder Cancer. European Urology. 2020 Apr 1;77(4):420-433.

[17] McConkey DJ, Choi W, Ochoa A, Dinney CP. Intrinsic subtypes and bladder cancer metastasis. Asian Journal of Urology. 2016 Oct;3(4): 260-267.

[18] Zhu S, Yu W, Yang X, Wu C, Cheng F. Traditional Classification and Novel Subtyping Systems for Bladder Cancer. Front Oncol. 2020 Feb 7;10:102-102.

[19] Volkmer J-P, Sahoo D, Chin RK, Ho PL, Tang C, Kurtova AV, et al. Three differentiation states risk-stratify bladder cancer into distinct subtypes. Proc Natl Acad Sci U S A. 2012/01/19 ed. 2012 Feb 7;109(6):2078-83.

[20] Hedegaard J, Lamy P, Nordentoft I, Algaba F, Høyer S, Ulhøi BP, et al. Comprehensive Transcriptional Analysis of Early-Stage Urothelial Carcinoma. Cancer Cell. 2016 Jul 11;30(1):27-42.

[21] van Kessel KEM, van der Keur KA, Dyrskjøt L, Algaba F, Welvaart NYC, Beukers W, et al. Molecular Markers Increase Precision of the European Association of Urology Non–Muscle-Invasive Bladder Cancer Progression Risk Groups. Clin Cancer Res. 2018 Apr 1;24(7):1586.

[22] Tan TZ, Rouanne M, Tan KT, Huang RY-J, Thiery J-P. Molecular Subtypes of Urothelial Bladder Cancer: Results from a Meta-cohort Analysis of 2411 Tumors. European Urology. 2019 Mar 1;75(3):423-432.

[23] Lerner SP, McConkey DJ, Hoadley KA, Chan KS, Kim WY, Radvanyi F, et al. Bladder Cancer Molecular Taxonomy: Summary from a Consensus Meeting. Bladder Cancer. 2016 Jan 7;2(1):37-47.

[24] Dadhania V, Zhang M, Zhang L, Bondaruk J, Majewski T, Siefker-Radtke A, et al. Meta-Analysis of the Luminal and Basal Subtypes of Bladder Cancer and the Identification of Signature Immunohistochemical Markers for Clinical Use. EBioMedicine. 2016 Aug 25;12:105-117.

[25] Seiler R, Gibb EA, Wang NQ, Oo HZ, Lam H-M, van Kessel KE, et al. Divergent Biological Response to Neoadjuvant Chemotherapy in Muscle-invasive Bladder Cancer. Clin Cancer Res. 2019 Aug 15;25(16):5082.

[26] Nogova L, Sequist LV, Perez Garcia JM, Andre F, Delord J-P, Hidalgo M, et al. Evaluation of BGJ398, a Fibroblast Growth Factor Receptor 1-3 Kinase Inhibitor, in Patients With Advanced Solid Tumors Harboring Genetic Alterations in Fibroblast Growth Factor Receptors: Results of a Global Phase I, Dose-Escalation and Dose-Expansion Study. JCO. 2016 Nov 21;35(2):157-165.

[27] Karkera JD, Cardona GM, Bell K, Gaffney D, Portale JC, Santiago-Walker A, et al. Oncogenic Characterization and Pharmacologic Sensitivity of Activating Fibroblast Growth Factor Receptor (FGFR) Genetic Alterations to the Selective FGFR Inhibitor Erdafitinib. Mol Cancer Ther. 2017 Aug 1;16(8):1717.

[28] Hoffman KL, Lerner SP, Smith CL. Raloxifene inhibits growth of RT4 urothelial carcinoma cells via estrogen receptor-dependent induction of apoptosis and inhibition of proliferation. Hormones & cancer. 2013;4:24-35

[29] Rosenberg JE, Hoffman-Censits J, Powles T, et al. Atezolizumab in patients with locally advanced and metastatic urothelial carcinoma who have

progressed following treatment with platinum-based chemotherapy: a single-arm, multicentre, phase 2 trial. Lancet. 2016;387:1909-1920.

[30] Esserman LJ, Berry DA, DeMichele A, Carey L, Davis SE, Buxton M, Hudis C, Gray JW, Perou C, Yau C, et al. Pathologic complete response predicts recurrence-free survival more effectively by cancer subset: results from the I-SPY 1 TRIAL--CALGB 150007/150012, ACRIN 6657. Journal of clinical oncology: official journal of the American Society of Clinical Oncology. 2012b;30:3242-3249

[31] Warrick JI, Sjödahl G, Kaag M, Raman JD, Merrill S, Shuman L, et al. Intratumoral Heterogeneity of Bladder Cancer by Molecular Subtypes and Histologic Variants. Eur Urol. 2019;75(1):18-22.

[32] Jangir H, Nambirajan A, Seth A, Sahoo RK, Dinda AK, Nayak B, et al. Prognostic stratification of muscle invasive urothelial carcinomas using limited immunohistochemical panel of Gata3 and cytokeratins 5/6, 14 and 20. Annals of Diagnostic Pathology. 2019 Dec;43:151397.

[33] Sjödahl G, Jackson CL, Bartlett JM, Siemens DR, Berman DM. Molecular profiling in muscle-invasive bladder cancer: more than the sum of its parts. The Journal of Pathology. 2019 Apr 1;247(5):563-573.

[34] Vale CL. Neoadjuvant Chemotherapy in Invasive Bladder Cancer: Update of a Systematic Review and Meta-Analysis of Individual Patient Data: Advanced Bladder Cancer (ABC) Meta-analysis Collaboration. European Urology. 2005 Aug 1;48(2):202-206.

[35] Krabbe L-M, Westerman ME, Margulis V, Raj G, Sagalowsky AI, Courtney KD, et al. Changing trends in utilization of neoadjuvant chemotherapy in muscle-invasive bladder cancer. JCO. 2014 May 20;32(15_suppl):e15518–e15518.

[36] Reardon ZD, Patel SG, Zaid HB, Stimson CJ, Resnick MJ, Keegan KA, et al. Trends in the use of perioperative chemotherapy for localized and locally advanced muscle-invasive bladder cancer: a sign of changing tides. Eur Urol. 2014/01/23 ed. 2015 Jan;67(1):165-70.

[37] Warrick JI, Knowles MA, Yves A, van der Kwast T, Grignon DJ, Kristiansen G, et al. Report From the International Society of Urological Pathology (ISUP) Consultation Conference On Molecular Pathology Of Urogenital Cancers. II. Molecular Pathology of Bladder Cancer: Progress and Challenges. The American Journal of Surgical Pathology. 2020 Jul;44(7):e30.

[38] Zeng S-X, Zhu Y, Ma A-H, Yu W, Zhang H, Lin T-Y, et al. The Phosphatidylinositol 3-Kinase Pathway as a Potential Therapeutic Target in Bladder Cancer. Clin Cancer Res. 2017/08/14 ed. 2017 Nov 1;23(21):6580-91.

[39] Powles T, Eder JP, Fine GD, Braiteh FS, Loriot Y, Cruz C, et al. MPDL3280A (anti-PD-L1) treatment leads to clinical activity in metastatic bladder cancer. Nature. 2014 Nov 1;515(7528):558-562.

[40] Aggen DH, Drake CG. Biomarkers for immunotherapy in bladder cancer: a moving target. J Immunother Cancer. 2017;5(1):94. Published 2017 Nov 21. doi:10.1186/s40425-017-0299-1

[41] Hodgson A, Slodkowska E, Jungbluth A, Liu SK, Vesprini D, Enepekides D, et al. PD-L1 immunohistochemistry assay concordance in urothelial carcinoma of the bladder and hypopharyngeal squamous cell carcinoma. Am J Surg Pathol. 2018 Aug;42(8):1059-1066.

[42] Zhu J, Armstrong AJ, Friedlander TW, Kim W, Pal SK, George DJ, et al. Biomarkers of immunotherapy in urothelial and renal cell carcinoma: PD-L1, tumor mutational burden, and beyond. Journal for Immunotherapy of Cancer. 2018;6:4.

[43] Balar AV, Galsky MD, Rosenberg JE, Powles T, Petrylak DP, Bellmunt J, et al. Atezolizumab as first-line treatment in cisplatin-ineligible patients with locally advanced and metastatic urothelial carcinoma: a single-arm, multicentre, phase 2 trial. Lancet. 2016/12/08 ed. 2017 Jan 7;389(10064):67-76.

Chapter 2

Bladder Cancer Variant Histologies: Epidemiology, Diagnosis, Treatment and Prognosis

Pedro Ramos, Pedro Pereira, Paulo Dinis and Luís Pacheco-Figueiredo

Abstract

Bladder cancer (BC) is an increasingly frequent cancer worldwide, being currently the sixth most frequent tumor and the thirteenth leading cause of cancer death. Among all BC cases, pathologists have identified several histomorphologies different from the conventional urothelial carcinoma. Although rare, these histologic variants have a distinct growth pattern, an altered cell differentiation and an unusual clinical behavior, especially concerning clinical presentation at diagnosis, response to the standard treatment and prognosis. Therefore, an updated review of this topic should be useful to aid clinicians in a better evidence-based decision-making. This chapter aims to summarize the current literature on the most common histologic variants regarding their epidemiology, clinical presentation at diagnosis, treatment options and prognosis. This includes both non-muscle invasive BC and muscle invasive BC as well as metastatic disease. A special focus will be placed on the role of neoadjuvant chemotherapy and early cystectomy and its prognostic implications.

Keywords: Bladder, Cancer, Histologic, Variants, Prognosis, Treatment

1. Introduction

Bladder cancer is an entity characterized by a wide range of different histomorphologies as well as distinct clinical courses. Approximately 75% of tumors are classified as pure urothelial carcinoma (transitional cell carcinoma), the remaining 25% consist of other histological variants. Several histological variants have been identified throughout the years, based on morphological features [1]. During the past decade, there is a trend of increasing evidence of the clinical relevance of histological variants, some them with data showing adverse pathological features and poor prognosis [2]. The acknowledgment of this information has been changing the clinical reasoning and disease management in patients with BC.

Pure non-urothelial bladder cancer comprises only a small minority (about 5%) of all bladder cancers. They include squamous cell carcinoma, adenocarcinoma, small cell carcinoma, and mixed histology tumors, with squamous and adenocarcinoma comprising the most frequent morphologies. Non-urothelial histologic subtypes were generally thought to have a worse prognosis compared to urothelial

IntechOpen

BC [3], however, once corrected for stage and patient-related factors, a significant proportion of them may have a similar prognosis.

On other hand, urothelial tumors with a variant histology component are more frequent than non-urothelial tumours. The classification of histologic variants is mainly based on morphologic features, being each differentiation pattern characterized by a distinct biological behavior, such as propensity for local recurrence and metastasis [4]. Non-muscle invasive BC with variant histology most likely remains underdiagnosed, as it seems challenging to identify its presence on TURB specimens. Current data suggests that variant histologies confer high-risk status to non-muscle invasive tumors, despite some studies had demonstrated similar progression rates in comparison with pure urothelial carcinomas (UC) associated with high risk factors [5]. Therefore, the question arises, does variant histology justify an aggressive treatment approach with early radical cystectomy?

The treatment of BC has evolved throughout the years such that clinical markers of risk are now used to guide us through algorithms that incorporate transurethral surgery, intravesical chemotherapy and immunotherapy, radical cystectomy, systemic combination chemotherapy, and sometimes radiation therapy. Therefore, the optimal risk stratification may include variant histology as a relevant factor in clinical decision making [6].

This chapter focuses on most common histological variants and discusses different treatment options and their prognostic value.

2. Histologic variants of Urothelial Carcinoma

Urothelial carcinoma (UC) is remarkable for displaying a wide range of diversity in its morphological appearance, which may reflect its molecular heterogeneity. Urothelial tumors with divergent differentiation are the most common histology variant within urothelial carcinomas [7]. The term refers to tumors that present some degree of typical urothelial carcinoma (invasive or *in situ*) with other histomorphologies such as squamous or glandular differentiation.

Squamous and Glandular differentiation are most common histology variants [8, 9]. UCs with squamous or glandular differentiation are distinct entities and should be distinguished from both pure squamous cell carcinoma (SCC) and or adenocarcinoma (AC) which do not include any urothelial components and subsequently present different clinical behavior. Other subtypes of UC variants include rarer differentiations including trophoblastic and small cell differentiation.

Urothelial carcinomas with divergent differentiation were previously thought to present at a more advanced stage at diagnosis and early reports indicated a poorer survival rate. More recently, studies have shown that, if standardized for stage, patients with either squamous or glandular UCs have survival rates comparable with those with pure UC.

Yet, current guidelines still categorize UC with variant histology in the highest risk category in which early radical cystectomy should be considered [8].

2.1 Urothelial carcinomas with squamous differentiation

Urothelial carcinomas with squamous differentiation are found in up to 40% of UCs and the inclusion of keratinization and/or intercellular bodies (**Figure 1**) are their main histological hallmarks [7]. The distinction between UC with squamous differentiation and pure squamous cell carcinomas (SCC) of the bladder remains a challenge for pathologists, especially in transurethral resection (TUR) specimens, because both tend to share most of the same immunohistochemical components.

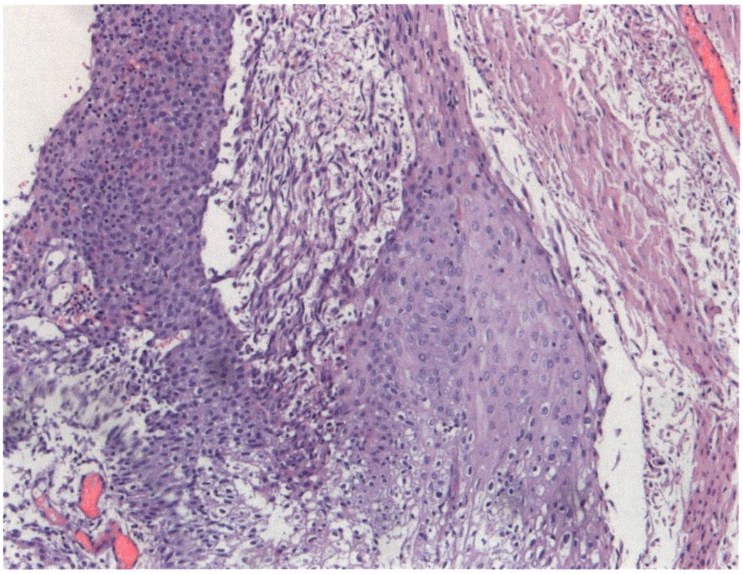

Figure 1.
Squamous differentiation is characterized by the presence of both urothelial carcinoma and keratin clusters and intercellular bodies (HE × 100).

Among NMIBC cases, UCs with squamous differentiation are frequently associated with high-grade and high-stage tumors at diagnosis and tend to have a less favorable response to intravesical chemotherapy or BCG instillations [10]. In the MIBC disease setting, studies have shown that response rate of neoadjuvant chemotherapy may be similar to conventional UC [11], although with a poor prognosis [2].

2.2 Urothelial carcinomas with glandular differentiation

Glandular differentiation comprises approximately 10% of all UCs and is characterized by true gland formation (**Figure 2**), resembling colonic adenocarcinoma, signet ring carcinoma or mucinous/colloid carcinoma. It may be associated with UC in situ or less frequently with in situ UC with glandular differentiation. Pseudo glandular aspects with mucin expression may be observed in conventional UC and should not be confused with either UC with glandular differentiation or bladder adenocarcinoma, although the lack of immunohistochemical markers makes the distinction challenging [12]. Telomerase reverse transcriptase (TERT) mutations are seen in the majority of UCs with glandular differentiation and not in adenocarcinomas of the bladder [13]; nevertheless, this marker is yet to be implemented in routine clinical use.

In terms of clinical significance of this differentiation, it tends to present at a higher stage, but it is not a predictor of adverse prognosis in stage-matched patients, showing similar rates of recurrence-free and overall survival when compared to conventional UC [5].

It is important to note that data from studies has showed that intravesical BCG treatment might play a key role in patients with UC with glandular differentiation, with this therapy presenting reasonable response rates [14, 15].

2.3 Urothelial Carcinomas with Trophoblastic Differentiation

UC with trophoblastic differentiation is a rare entity with only a few cases reported, and it is characterized by the expression of the beta subunit of the human chorionic gonadotropin (ßhCG) (**Figure 3**). This subtype must be distinguished from

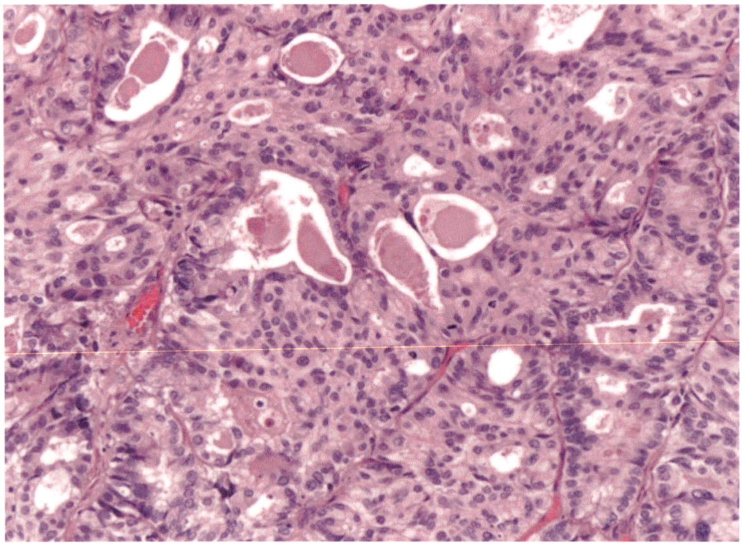

Figure 2.
Glandular differentiation encompasses gland-like lumina or fully developed adenocarcinoma with intestinal morphology (HE × 100).

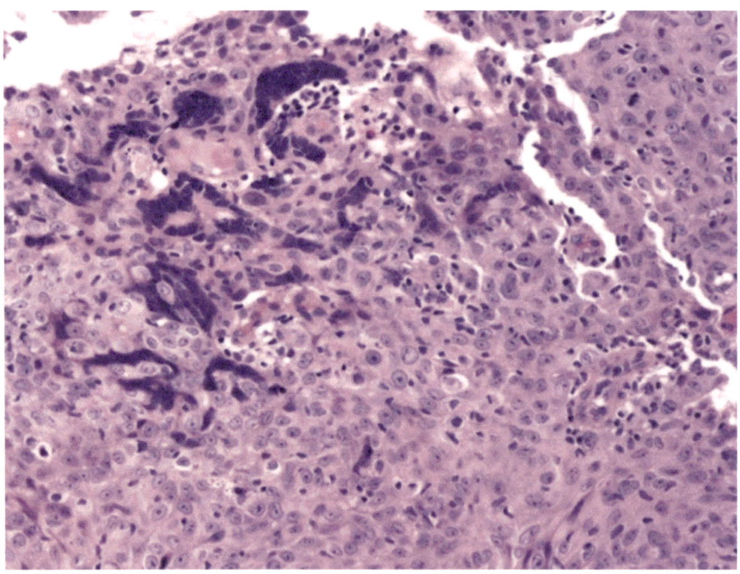

Figure 3.
The image shows a cluster of syncytiotrophoblastic giant cells enclosed by high-grade urothelial carcinoma (HE × 100).

pure choriocarcinoma which requires the demonstration of the isochromosome 12p, a hallmark of germ cell tumors. The percentage of ßhCG-immunoreactive cells is associated with higher stage and grade of the disease. Elevated secretion of ßhCG into the serum may be associated with an observable poorer response to chemotherapy and radiation, and it can be used as a marker in the follow-up of these patients [2].

2.4 Urothelial Carcinomas with Small Cell Differentiation

UC can exhibit neuroendocrine differentiation in the form of small cell carcinoma. These tumors are usually treated similarly to their counterpart in the lungs.

2.5 Nested Urothelial Carcinoma

Based on the 2016 WHO classification, the nested variant includes UC with small tubules and microcysts (**Figure 4**). This histologic variant can often resemble benign cytology [16]. It is characterized by disorderly proliferation of confluent nests, with minimal cell atypia [17], which can often delay the definitive diagnosis.

Nested UCs usually present as high stage disease and may be associated with a worse prognosis compared with pure nested variants [14]. It shares similar immunohistochemical features and clinical outcomes with the conventional UC, with little to no difference in recurrence rate or survival when treated with RC in either NMIBC and MIBC [17].

2.6 Microcystic Urothelial Carcinoma

The microcystic UC variant, like the nested UCs, is characterized by a benign cytologic resemblance features. It is constituted by oval cysts, lined by urothelial, low columnar or flattened epithelium (**Figure 5**) and focal conventional UC may be present in up to 40% of tumors [18]. Foci of high-grade UC are seen in up to 40% of cases, which may help distinguish this variant form benign mimicking tumors [14].

Differential diagnosis includes benign proliferations such as florid polypoid cystitis cystica and glanduraris and adenocarcinoma [19].

There is very limited information about prognostic implications of microcystic histology in BC, only a few case reports and case series have been published. The largest study to date (N = 20) reported 55% of patients died at a mean follow-up of 30 months after radical cystectomy (RC). However, when controlled for stage, there was no statistically significant difference in survival compared with patients with pure UC [20].

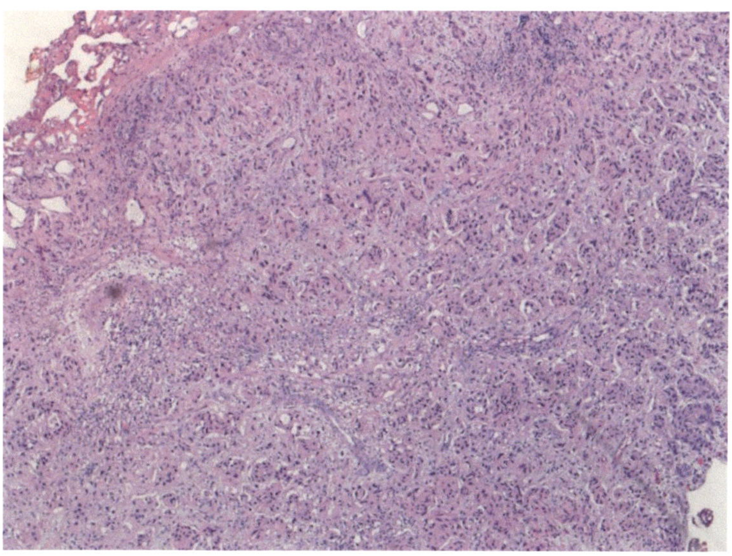

Figure 4.
The nested variant of urothelial carcinoma consists of small, discrete nests with bland morphology distributed irregularly in the lamina propria. The size of nests is much smaller than von Brunn's nests of normal urothelium (HE × 40).

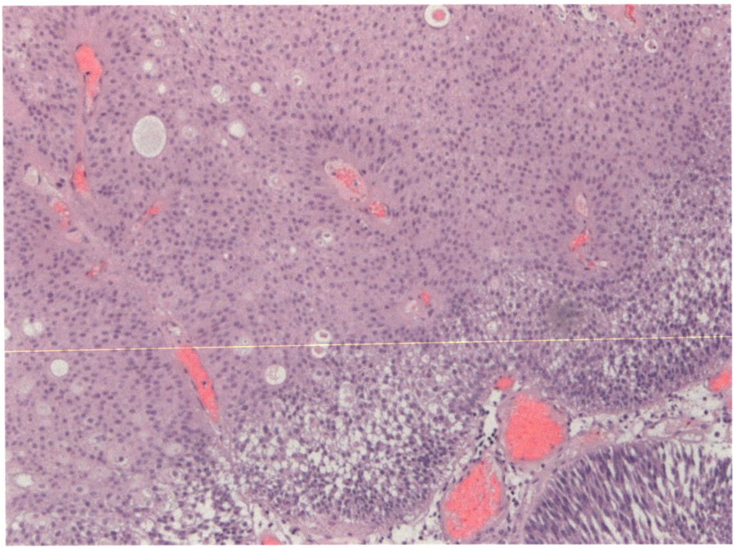

Figure 5.
Characterized by the formation of microcysts which may mimic cystitis cystica in small specimens. Cytologic atypia is minimal or entirely absent (HE × 100).

2.7 Micropapillary Urothelial Carcinoma

Micropapillary Urothelial Carcinoma (MPUC) is a variant seen most commonly in males, being characterized by small tumour nests surrounded by lacunar spaces (**Figure 6**). It is a clinically aggressive variant that usually presents at an advanced stage that accounts for 2–5% of UCs [14, 21]. ERBB2 (HER2) amplification by FISH is seen more commonly in patients with MPUC versus conventional UC, such expression has been related to worse cancer-specific survival although it also provides a potential role for HER2 targeted therapy [22]. Single institution case-series

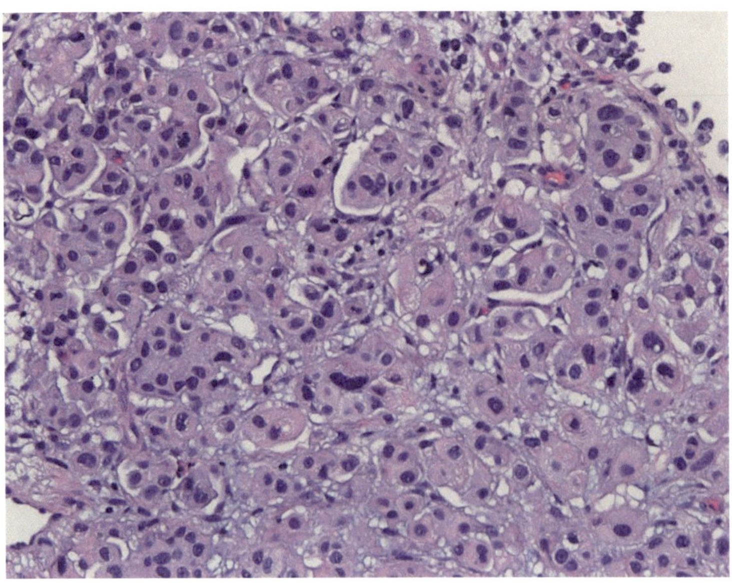

Figure 6.
Infiltrating tumors cells with slender filiform processes without fibrovascular cores and multiple small tumor nests within a single lacunar space, mostly not enclosing a true fibrovascular core (HE × 200).

have demonstrated poorer outcomes in patients with MPUC than those with pure UC [23]. However, more recent studies demonstrated that, when controlled for stage, this may not be the case.

Non muscle-invasive MPUC is characterized by high rates of progression to muscle-invasive and metastatic BC. A case series with 44 patients with non-muscle invasive MPUC, amongst those treated with BCG, 67% showed cancer progression with 22% developing metastatic disease, only 19% remained alive at the end of follow-up (10-yeat) without RC. Patients who underwent delayed RC after BCG treatment failure presented a median disease-specific survival (DSS) of 62% at 10 years. On the other hand, patients treated with early RC had a 10-year median DSS of 72% [24].

Patients with UC with a micropapillary component doing upfront RC were not associated with worse recurrence-free, cancer specific or overall survival, when compared to those with pure UC [25].

Therefore, early RC has been considered the standard of care in most centers, however, there have been reports of reasonable outcomes in series in which bladder preservation therapies were applied in highly selected patients with a relatively small micropapillary component [26].

Although there is still scarce evidence regarding muscle-invasive MPUC and the role of Neo-adjuvant chemotherapy (NAC) in opposition to early RC, there have been reports showing no statistically significant differences in overall survival (OS) between the group who have undergone NAC plus RC vs. RC only [27]. A recent study analyzed the impact of adjuvant chemotherapy (AC) in the OS among patients with MPUC and the results demonstrated that, in contrast to pure UC, no survival benefit was observed in patients with this histology subtype [28]. Nevertheless, although these results could be explained by the more aggressive clinical behavior of this histologic variant, they can also be a consequence of small samples size, short follow-up periods and lack of risk stratification in most studies.

2.8 Lymphoepithelioma-like UC

Lymphoepithelioma-like UC (LLUC) resembles lymphoepithelioma of the nasopharynx and is characterized by a prominent lymphoid stroma (**Figure** 7) with T (predominantly CD3) and B lymphocytes, plasma cells, histiocytes, neutrophils and eosinophils. Major differential diagnosis comprises poorly differentiated UC with lymphoid inflammatory response or lymphoma [29, 30].

This histologic variant has been found to have a similar prognosis to conventional UC as well as similar chemosensitivity and response to immunotherapy [31].

2.9 Plasmocytoid

Plasmacytoid UC is a rare histopathological variant of UC, comprising 1–3% of all UCs and is characterized by the presence of discohesive cells with eccentrically placed nuclei surrounded by abundant eosinophilic cytoplasm (**Figure 8**). This variant usually displays a diffusely infiltrative growth pattern, inducing minimal stromal reaction [32]. This morphology is not exclusive to UC, thus plasmacytoid UC (PUC) must be distinguished from melanoma and lymphoma. Immunohistochemical markers such as CK7, CK20 uroplakin II, and GATA-3 can be useful in the differentiation in doubtful situations [33]. It is also characterized by a distinct growth pattern in which tumour cells can manifest distant from macroscopic disease with the absence of a desmoplastic reaction making it more challenging to determine the plane between the tumour and normal tissue. A wide margin of resection is therefore mandatory to ensure an adequate resection at the time of RC [32].

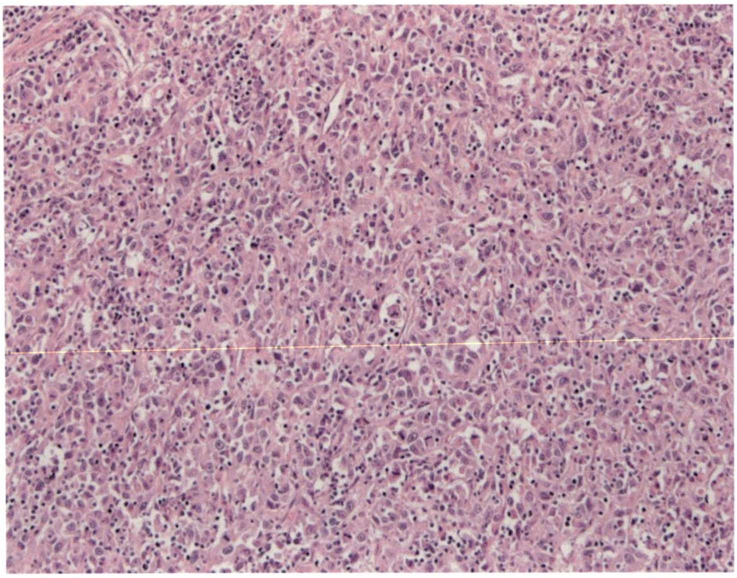

Figure 7.
Characterized by syncytial sheets of tumor cells and a prominent chronic inflammatory infiltrate in the stroma. The infiltrate is composed largely of lymphocytes, plasma cells, eosinophils, and other inflammatory cells which may create an appearance of chronic cystitis or malignant lymphoma (HE × 100).

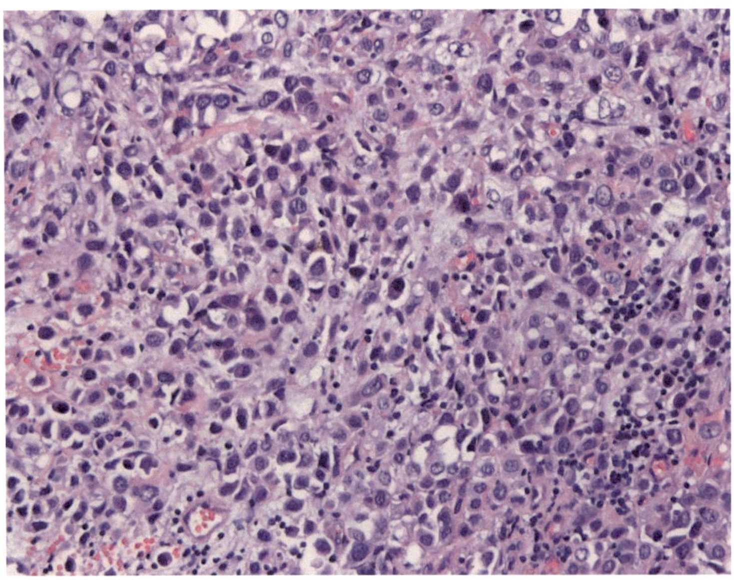

Figure 8.
PUC usually displays single tumor cells with plasmacytoid features infiltrating loose myxoid stroma. It shows discohesive tumour cells with eccentrically located nuclei and abundant eosinophilic cytoplasm (HE × 200).

Mutations in CDH1 are pathognomonic of PUC and result in the loss of E-cadherin expression in its tumour cells, this is thought to explain the higher rates of tumour cell migration observed [34, 35].

Plasmacytoid UC response to intravesical BCG has not been clearly defined yet but given the fact that these tumors display a strong predilection for recurrence, especially in peritoneal lining, even in cases when non-muscle invasiveness is encountered, early RC seems to provide a more effective control of the disease [36].

The role of NAC/AC is still unclear in PUC, although initial evidence suggested this histologic variant was chemosensitive, more recent data suggests that platin based regimens confer no survival enhancement and that even in patients who achieve pT0 stage after cystectomy after RC, poor prognosis is maintained in PUC [36, 37].

2.10 Sarcomatoid

Sarcomatoid UC accounts for approximately 0.3% of all UCs. This histologic variant is characterized highly variable morphology exhibiting both epithelial and mesenchymal differentiation with high-grade spindle cells (**Figure 9**). Previous exposure to radiotherapy (RT) and intravesical cyclophosphamide are known risk factors [38].

Sarcomatoid differentiation has been associated with a very poor prognosis, since it usually presents at an advanced stage [38]. However recent series demonstrated no differences in comparison with same stage pure UC, regarding disease-specific, all-cause mortality and overall survival [28]. A survival benefit was not found in patients undergoing NAC or AC, suggesting this variant might be particularly resistant to chemotherapy [39].

2.11 Clear cell

Clear cell UC is a very rare variant of UC characterized by tumour cells with glycogen-rich cytoplasm (**Figure 10**). It is crucial to do the correct differential diagnosis among clear cell UC, clear cell adenocarcinoma of the bladder, metastatic clear cell renal cell carcinoma or clear cell carcinoma of the female genital tract [28].

Only a few case reports are available for this rare histologic variant. The evidence suggests a high progression rate to muscle-invasive and metastatic BC, and although treatment strategy is poorly defined, an aggressive approach with early RC is advocated [40].

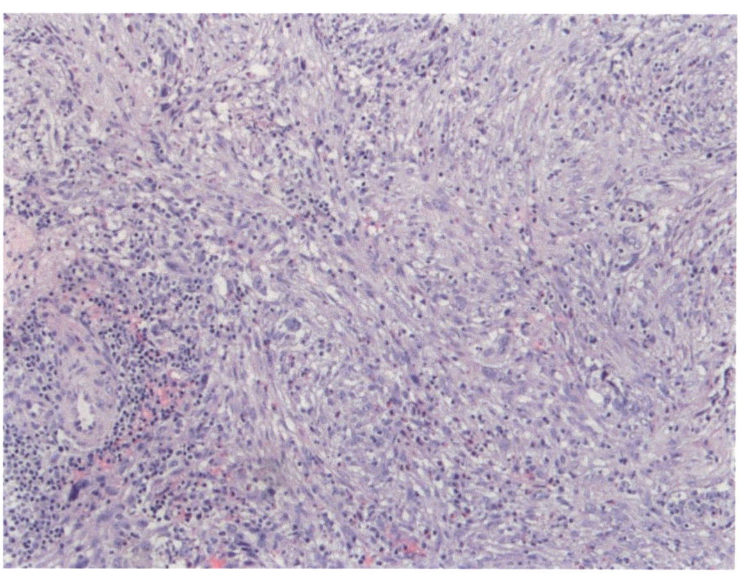

Figure 9.
It contains both carcinoma as well as sarcomatous areas usually with high-grade urothelial carcinoma on the surface and a high-grade undifferentiated sarcoma underneath in the lamina propria (HE × 100).

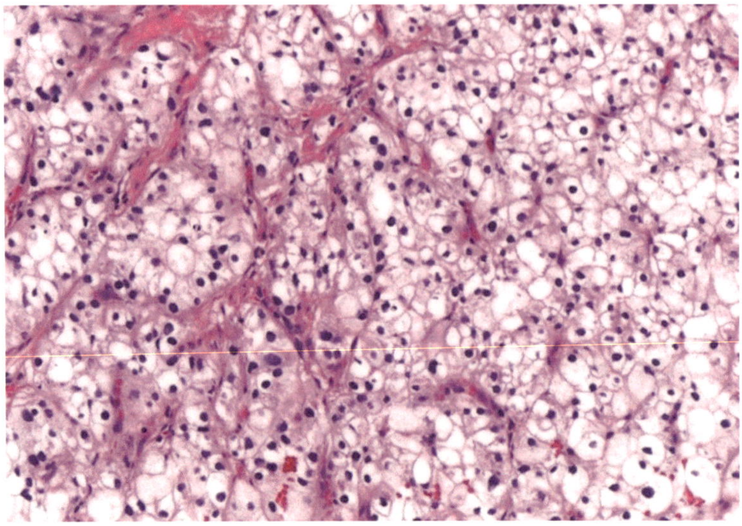

Figure 10.
Clear cell variant of urothelial carcinoma consists of abundant clear cytoplasm due to glycogen content and it is characterized by large nests of tumour cells with high- grade nuclear atypia and clear cytoplasm (HE × 200).

3. Non-Urothelial Variants

Non-urothelial BC can be categorized as epithelial and non-epithelial tumors. Approximately 90% are epithelial, including squamous cell carcinoma, adenocarcinoma and small-cell carcinoma. Non-epithelial tumors are rare, and include sarcoma, corinosarcoma, paraganglioma, melanoma and lymphoma [41]. In this section we will restrict our description to the most common subtypes.

4. Squamous Cell Carcinoma

Squamous Cell Carcinoma (SCC) represents the most common non-urothelial histologic variant, accounting for almost 2–5% of all BC in the western world and approximately 30% in endemic regions (Egypt and other parts of Africa) due to the parasite *Schistosoma haematobium* infection, which causes bilharzial SCC [42]. Non-bilharzial SCC is associated with chronic inflammation of the urothelium as a result of chronic urinary tract infection, long-term indwelling catheters and bladder calculi. In contrast to UC, the relationship between SCC and cigarette smoking in not clearly established [43].

In terms of histological characteristics, SCC contains keratin pearl inclusions and granules (**Figure 11**). Moreover, microscopic analysis shows that most SCC tumors are moderately to poorly differentiated tumors.

SCC tends to appear in the seventh decade of life, except for spinal cord injured patients which can present at younger ages and is characterized by a slight male predominance with a higher proportion of non-Caucasians [44]. SCC is associated with more advanced disease at presentation compared to UC, with 70% of cases showing muscle-invasiveness at time of diagnosis, with a higher propensity for nodal involvement and metastatic disease [45]. Even in patients with T1 staging at diagnosis, pure SCC has been identified as an independent predictor of mortality in patients who did not undergo early cystectomy [46]. However, data from studies has also reported that, in cases in which the tumor was confined to the bladder wall and the bladder was surgically removed as part of the initial treatment, SCC histologic features were not associated with increased mortality when compared to UC [41, 47].

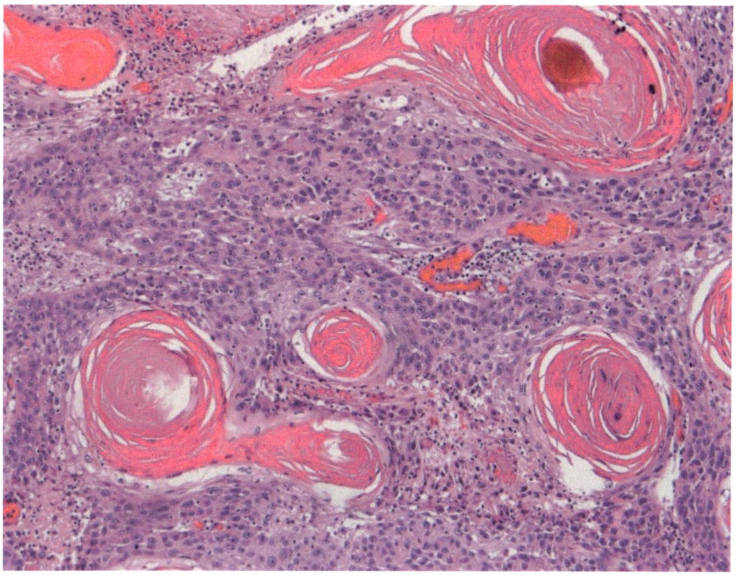

Figure 11.
The image shows presence of keratin pearls and copious keratin production, unequivocal for squamous differentiation (HE × 100).

This histological subtype has been associated with poorer OS, even when adjusted for stage. However, bilharzial-associated SCC, which usually presents at a younger age, is associated with lower stages at diagnosis, and a more indolent disease course with subsequent better survival outcomes [48].

In opposition to UC, NAC has not demonstrated a statistically significant improvement in OS among patients with the SCC histology, treated with RC [49].

Regarding radiation therapy, there is some evidence that treatment with pre-operative RT may improve disease-free survival comparing with RC alone [49]. Moreover, since SCC histology subtype is notoriously chemo-resistant to most regiments used for metastatic UC, radiotherapy can have an important therapeutic role [50]. This data was, however, obtained from retrospective studies with a very limited number of cases, suggesting that conclusions must be further evaluated.

Based on the best published evidence, early RC remains the mainstay therapy in patients with high-risk SCC, even when non-muscle invasive staging is observed [28]. It is important to note that, unlike other histologic subtypes, pelvic lymph node dissection (PLND) was associated with an improvement in OS [51].

5. Adenocarcinoma

Adenocarcinoma (AC) of the bladder can be primary or secondary [if it results from a contiguous invasion from other organs such as prostate, colon or uterus (endometrium and cervix), or metastatic spread (lung)]. Primary AC accounts for roughly 2% of all BCs and is divided into two subtypes: Urachal (10%) and nonurachal AC. There are also different types of adenocarcinomas that have been described, including glandular (**Figure 12**), colloid, papillary, signet ring and clear cell. Known risk factors include bilharziasis, chronic inflammation and bladder exstrophy (even in patients who have undergone correction in the neonatal period) [43, 51]. The diagnosis of primary AC of the bladder should only be made if secondary involvement from other organs is excluded. This entity has been shown to be more common in females, with a higher proportion among non-caucasians [52].

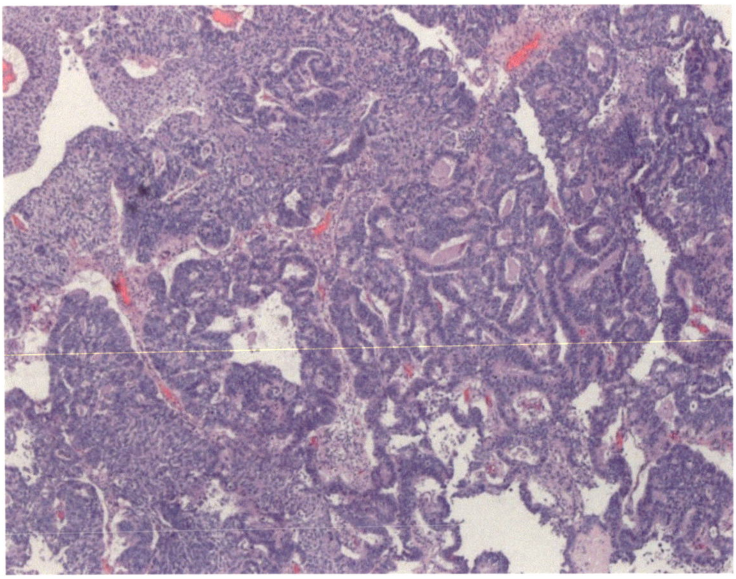

Figure 12.
Intestinal-type adenocarcinoma shows malignant colonic glands with high-grade columnar cells and necrosis in the lumens (HE × 40).

Bladder AC usually presents at an advanced stage, with muscle-invasive or metastatic disease. For localized disease, RC is currently the treatment of choice. However, when matched for stage, primary AC appears to have similar outcomes to UC [53]. In patients with NMIBC disease, a SEER analysis reports that, in non-urachal AC, transurethral resection (TUR) alone increased mortality risk, compared with early cystectomy [54]. There is currently no evidence available regarding the effect of immuno- or chemotherapy.

Urachal AC seems to present more favorable prognosis compared with non-urachal AC. Partial cystectomy (with en bloc resection of the bladder dome and umbilical ligament) is an alternative option to RC, in selected patients [55, 56]. Although urachal AC also seems more likely to present as metastatic disease in comparison to UC, the previous mentioned better prognosis is most probably partly due to be diagnosed among younger patients, with less co-morbidities [28].

Current data about NAC or AC in adenocarcinoma patients, although very scarce, suggests that neither therapy confers an improvement in survival [57].

5.1 Small Cell Carcinoma

The urinary bladder is the most common site for genitourinary extra-pulmonary neuroendocrine/small cell carcinomas. Small cell carcinoma (SmCC) accounts for less than 1% of BCs. It is a neuroendocrine tumour characterized by nests or solid sheets of small cells with enlarged nuclei, evenly dispersed chromatin with a "salt and pepper" pattern (**Figure 13**), with abundant resemblance to its pulmonary counterpart. It often co-exists with conventional UC, SCC and AC. Neuroendocrine markers such as chromogranin, synaptophysin and CD56 are expressed in SmCC [43]. Mean age presentation sits in the seventh-decade of life, with a strong male predominance (5:1) [55]. SmCC also shows similar characteristics to small cell carcinomas of the lung including ectopic hormone production, which can lead to clinically relevant hyperkalemia and hypophosphatemia [56, 58].

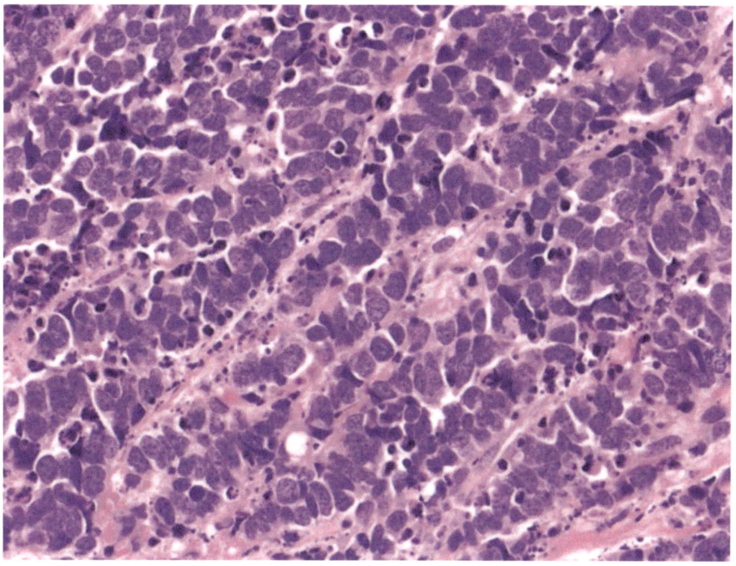

Figure 13.
Small cells with artifacts that make it difficult to distinguish between cytoplasm and nucleus (HE × 100).

This histologic variant is also characterized by its aggressiveness, exhibiting rapid growth with a predilection for early metastases, and a particularly high propensity for brain metastasis [59].

Contrarily to many of other histologic variants, a treatment strategy based on NAC followed by RC or RT represents the optimal strategy, based on several studies that demonstrated the chemosensitivity (with platinum-based therapy) of SmCC with an improvement in survival [59].

In terms of prognosis, SmCC presents a similar outcome to pure UC at same stages, except in the setting of diffuse metastatic disease in which it presents worse outcomes [60].

6. Conclusions

Bladder cancer with UC variants and non-urothelial subtypes have been classically described as tumors with a worse prognosis in comparison with pure UCs. However, the latter is mostly explained by a higher stage at the diagnosis among non-pure UC, since data from case-series and retrospective studies seems to suggest that, among the majority of variants, the prognosis is similar to pure UC, after adjustment for the disease stage.

Current diagnosis of variant histology in BC provides clinically relevant information to the physician and a novel framework to stratify patients according to prognosis, risk of recurrence and expected response to a given therapy. However, the management of this conditions remains challenging. Currently, RC preceded, in some tumors by NAC, constitutes the recommended treatment approach for resecable disease; AC is most commonly unsuccessful and data on immunotherapy is still scant. Regarding immunotherapy, it appears that drugs active in the PD-1 pathway are independent of histology [60].

Additionally, molecular alterations unique to these variants could be of use, in the future, as targeted therapies could emerge as a treatment option. However, further investigation is still needed to understand more clearly the diagnostic criteria to be applied in these entities. Multicenter, international, prospective collaborative efforts are needed in order to clarify the distinct prognosis of these patients and to determine optimal therapy regimens.

Author details

Pedro Ramos[1]*, Pedro Pereira[2,4], Paulo Dinis[1,2] and Luís Pacheco-Figueiredo[1,3]

1 Urology Department, Centro Hospitalar e Universitário de São João, Porto, Portugal

2 Faculty of Medicine, University of Porto, Portugal

3 Life and Health Sciences Research Institute (ICVS), School of Medicine, University of Minho, Braga, Portugal

4 Pathology Department, Centro Hospitalar e Universitário de São João, Porto, Portugal

*Address all correspondence to: u015827@chsj.min-saude.pt

References

[1] Moschini M, D'Andrea D, Korn S, Irmak Y, Soria F, Compérat E, et al. Characteristics and clinical significance of histological variants of bladder cancer. Vol. 14, Nature Reviews Urology. Nature Publishing Group; 2017. p. 651-68.

[2] Lopez-Beltran A, Henriques V, Montironi R, Cimadamore A, Raspollini MR, Cheng L. Variants and new entities of bladder cancer. Vol. 74, Histopathology. Blackwell Publishing Ltd.; 2019. p. 77-96.

[3] Alanee S, Alvarado-Cabrero I, Murugan P, Kumar R, Nepple KG, Paner GP, et al. Update of the International Consultation on Urological Diseases on bladder cancer 2018: non-urothelial cancers of the urinary bladder. World Journal of Urology. 2019 Jan 23;37(1):107-14.

[4] Park S, Reuter VE, Hansel DE. Non-urothelial carcinomas of the bladder. Vol. 74, Histopathology. Blackwell Publishing Ltd.; 2019. p. 97-111.

[5] Shapur NK, Katz R, Pode D, Shapiro A, Yutkin V, Pizov G, et al. Is radical cystectomy mandatory in every patient with variant histology of bladder cancer. Rare Tumors. 2011 Apr 4;3(2):67-70.

[6] Black PC, Brown GA, Dinney CPN. The impact of variant histology on the outcome of bladder cancer treated with curative intent. Vol. 27, Urologic Oncology: Seminars and Original Investigations. 2009. p. 3-7.

[7] Compérat E, Gontero P, Mostafid AH, Palou J, van Rhijn BWG, Rouprêt M, et al. Non-muscle-invasive Bladder Cancer (TaT1 and CIS) EAU Guidelines on. 2020.

[8] Choi W, Porten S, Kim S, Willis D, Plimack ER, Hoffman-Censits J, et al. Identification of Distinct Basal and Luminal Subtypes of Muscle-Invasive Bladder Cancer with Different Sensitivities to Frontline Chemotherapy. Cancer Cell. 2014 Feb 10;25(2):152-65.

[9] Lagwinski N, Thomas A, Stephenson AJ, Campbell S, Hoschar AP, El-Gabry E, et al. Squamous Cell Carcinoma of the Bladder: A Clinicopathologic Analysis of 45 Cases. Vol. 31, Am J Surg Pathol. 2007.

[10] Veskimäe E, Espinos EL, Bruins HM, Yuan Y, Sylvester R, Kamat AM, et al. What Is the Prognostic and Clinical Importance of Urothelial and Nonurothelial Histological Variants of Bladder Cancer in Predicting Oncological Outcomes in Patients with Muscle-invasive and Metastatic Bladder Cancer? A European Association of Urology Muscle Invasive and Metastatic Bladder Cancer Guidelines Panel Systematic Review. European urology oncology. 2019 Nov 1;2(6):625-42.

[11] Baumeister P, Zamboni S, Mattei A, Antonelli A, Simeone C, Mordasini L, et al. Histological variants in non-muscle invasive bladder cancer. Vol. 8, Translational Andrology and Urology. AME Publishing Company; 2019. p. 34-8.

[12] Vail E, Zheng X, Zhou M, Yang X, Fallon JT, Epstein JI, et al. Telomerase reverse transcriptase promoter mutations in glandular lesions of the urinary bladder. Annals of Diagnostic Pathology. 2015 Oct 1;19(5):301-5.

[13] Kim SP, Frank I, Cheville JC, Thompson RH, Weight CJ, Thapa P, et al. The impact of squamous and glandular differentiation on survival after radical cystectomy for urothelial carcinoma. Journal of Urology. 2012 Aug;188(2):405-9.

[14] Lopez-Beltran A, Henriques V, Montironi R, Cimadamore A,

Raspollini MR, Cheng L. Variants and new entities of bladder cancer. Vol. 74, Histopathology. Blackwell Publishing Ltd.; 2019. p. 77-96.

[15] Douglas J, Sharp A, Chau C, Head J, Drake T, Wheater M, et al. Serum total hCGβ level is an independent prognostic factor in transitional cell carcinoma of the urothelial tract. British Journal of Cancer. 2014 Apr 1;110(7):1759-66.

[16] Warrick JI. Clinical significance of histologic variants of bladder cancer. Vol. 15, JNCCN Journal of the National Comprehensive Cancer Network. Harborside Press; 2017. p. 1268-74.

[17] Aron M. Variant Histology in Bladder Cancer—Current Understanding of Pathologic Subtypes. Vol. 20, Current Urology Reports. Springer; 2019.

[18] Lopez Beltran A, Montironi R, Cheng L. Microcystic urothelial carcinoma: Morphology, immunohistochemistry and clinical behaviour. Histopathology. 2014;64(6):872-9.

[19] amin1994.

[20] Sui W, Matulay JT, James MB, Onyeji IC, Theofanides MC, RoyChoudhury A, et al. Micropapillary bladder cancer: Insights from the national cancer database. Bladder Cancer. 2016;2(4):415-23.

[21] Schneider SA, Sukov WR, Frank I, Boorjian SA, Costello BA, Tarrell RF, et al. Outcome of patients with micropapillary urothelial carcinoma following radical cystectomy: ERBB2 (HER2) amplification identifies patients with poor outcome. Modern Pathology. 2014;27(5):758-64.

[22] Abufaraj M, Foerster B, Schernhammer E, Moschini M, Kimura S, Hassler MR, et al. Micropapillary Urothelial Carcinoma of the Bladder: A Systematic Review and Meta-analysis of Disease Characteristics and Treatment Outcomes. Vol. 75, European Urology. Elsevier B.V.; 2019. p. 649-58.

[23] Kamat AM, Dinney CPN, Gee JR, Grossman HB, Siefker-Radtke AO, Tamboli P, et al. Micropapillary bladder cancer: A review of the University of Texas M. D. Anderson Cancer Center experience with 100 consecutive patients. Cancer. 2007 Jul 1;110(1):62-7.

[24] Kamat AM, Gee JR, Dinney CPN, Grossman HB, Swanson DA, Millikan RE, et al. The case for early cystectomy in the treatment of nonmuscle invasive micropapillary bladder carcinoma. Journal of Urology. 2006;175(3):881-5.

[25] Vetterlein MW, Mullane S, Seisen T, Lander R, Löppenberg B, Choueiri TK, et al. MP34-11 NEOADJUVANT CHEMOTHERAPY PRIOR TO RADICAL CYSTECTOMY FOR MUSCLE-INVASIVE BLADDER CANCER WITH VARIANT HISTOLOGY. Journal of Urology. 2017 Apr;197(4S).

[26] Berg S, D'Andrea D, Vetterlein MW, Cole AP, Fletcher SA, Krimphove MJ, et al. Impact of adjuvant chemotherapy in patients with adverse features and variant histology at radical cystectomy for muscle-invasive carcinoma of the bladder: Does histologic subtype matter? Cancer. 2019 May 1;125(9):1449-58.

[27] Lobo N, Shariat SF, Guo CC, Fernandez MI, Kassouf W, Choudhury A, et al. What Is the Significance of Variant Histology in Urothelial Carcinoma? Vol. 6, European Urology Focus. Elsevier B.V.; 2020. p. 653-63.

[28] Lobo N, Shariat SF, Guo CC, Fernandez MI, Kassouf W, Choudhury A, et al. What Is the

Significance of Variant Histology in Urothelial Carcinoma? Vol. 6, European Urology Focus. Elsevier B.V.; 2020. p. 653-63.

[29] Tamas EF, Nielsen ME, Schoenberg MP, Epstein JI. Lymphoepithelioma-like carcinoma of the urinary tract: A clinicopathological study of 30 pure and mixed cases. Modern Pathology. 2007 Aug 11;20(8):828-34.

[30] Yang AW, Pooli A, Lele SM, Kim IW, Davies JD, LaGrange CA. Lymphoepithelioma-like, a variant of urothelial carcinoma of the urinary bladder: a case report and systematic review for optimal treatment modality for disease-free survival. BMC Urology. 2017 Apr 27;17(1).

[31] Fox MD, Xiao L, Zhang M, Kamat AM, Siefker-Radtke A, Zhang L, et al. Plasmacytoid Urothelial Carcinoma of the Urinary Bladder. Vol. 147, American Journal of Clinical Pathology. Oxford University Press; 2017. p. 500-6.

[32] Li Q, Assel M, Benfante NE, Pietzak EJ, Herr HW, Donat M, et al. The Impact of Plasmacytoid Variant Histology on the Survival of Patients with Urothelial Carcinoma of Bladder after Radical Cystectomy. European Urology Focus. 2019 Jan 1;5(1):104-8.

[33] Dayyani F, Czerniak BA, Sircar K, Munsell MF, Millikan RE, Dinney CP, et al. Plasmacytoid urothelial carcinoma, a chemosensitive cancer with poor prognosis, and peritoneal carcinomatosis. Journal of Urology. 2013;189(5):1656-61.

[34] Kaimakliotis HZ, Monn MF, Cheng L, Masterson TA, Cary KC, Pedrosa JA, et al. Plasmacytoid bladder cancer: Variant histology with aggressive behavior and a new mode of invasion along fascial planes. Urology. 2014;83(5):1112-6.

[35] Diamantopoulos LN, Khaki AR, Grivas P, Gore JL, Schade GR, Hsieh AC, et al. Plasmacytoid Urothelial Carcinoma: Response to Chemotherapy and Oncologic Outcomes. Bladder Cancer. 2020;6(1):71-81.

[36] Lopez-Beltran A, Pacelli A, Rothenberg HJ, Wollan PC, Zincke H, Blute ML, et al. CARCINOSARCOMA AND SARCOMATOID CARCINOMA OF THE BLADDER: CLINICOPATHOLOGICAL STUDY OF 41 CASES. Vol. 159, AMERICAN UROLOCICAL ASSOCIATION, INC. 1998.

[37] Wright JL, Black PC, Brown GA, Porter MP, Kamat AM, Dinney CP, et al. Differences in Survival Among Patients With Sarcomatoid Carcinoma, Carcinosarcoma and Urothelial Carcinoma of the Bladder. Journal of Urology. 2007 Dec;178(6):2302-7.

[38] Black PC, Brown GA, Dinney CPN. The impact of variant histology on the outcome of bladder cancer treated with curative intent. Vol. 27, Urologic Oncology: Seminars and Original Investigations. 2009. p. 3-7.

[39] Mihai I, Taban S, Cumpanas A, Olteanu EG, Iacob M, Dema A. Clear cell urothelial carcinoma of the urinary bladder - a rare pathological entity. A case report and a systematic review of the literature. Bosnian Journal of Basic Medical Sciences. 2019;19(4):400-3.

[40] Klaile Y, Schlack K, Boegemann M, Steinestel J, Schrader AJ, Krabbe LM. Variant histology in bladder cancer: How it should change the management in non-muscle invasive and muscle invasive disease? Vol. 5, Translational Andrology and Urology. AME Publishing Company; 2016. p. 692-701.

[41] Izard JP, Siemens DR, Mackillop WJ, Wei X, Leveridge MJ, Berman DM, et al. Outcomes of squamous histology in bladder cancer: A population-based

study. Urologic Oncology: Seminars and Original Investigations. 2015 Oct 1;33(10):425.e7-425.e13.

[42] Kantor AF, Hartge P, Hoover RN, Fraumeni JF. Epidemiological Characteristics of Squamous Cell Carcinoma and Adenocarcinoma of the Bladder1. Vol. 48, CANCER RESEARCH. 1988.

[43] Pons F, Orsola A, Morote J, Bellmunt J. Variant forms of bladder cancer: Basic considerations on treatment approaches. Current Oncology Reports. 2011 Jun;13(3):216-21.

[44] El-Sebaie M, Zaghloul MS, Howard G, Mokhtar A. Squamous cell carcinoma of the bilharzial and non-bilharzial urinary bladder: A review of etiological features, natural history, and management. Vol. 10, International Journal of Clinical Oncology. 2005. p. 20-5.

[45] Matulay JT, Woldu SL, Lim A, Narayan VM, Li G, Kamat AM, et al. The impact of squamous histology on survival in patients with muscle-invasive bladder cancer. Urologic Oncology: Seminars and Original Investigations. 2019 Jun 1;37(6):353.e17-353.e24.

[46] Scosyrev E, Yao J, Messing E. Urothelial Carcinoma Versus Squamous Cell Carcinoma of Bladder: Is Survival Different With Stage Adjustment? Urology. 2009 Apr;73(4):822-7.

[47] Zahoor H, Elson P, Stephenson A, Haber GP, Kaouk J, Fergany A, et al. Patient Characteristics, Treatment Patterns and Prognostic Factors in Squamous Cell Bladder Cancer. Clinical Genitourinary Cancer. 2018 Apr 1;16(2):e437-42.

[48] Porten SP, Willis D, Kamat AM. Variant histology: Role in management and prognosis of nonmuscle invasive bladder cancer. Vol. 24, Current Opinion in Urology. Lippincott Williams and Wilkins; 2014. p. 517-23.

[49] Serretta V, Pomara G, Piazza F, Gange E. Pure Squamous Cell Carcinoma of the Bladder in Western Countries. European Urology. 2000;37:85-9.

[50] Guo L, Zhang L, Wang J, Zhang X, Zhu Z. Pelvic Lymph Node Dissection During Cystectomy for Patients With Bladder Carcinoma With Variant Histology: Does Histologic Type Matter? Frontiers in Oncology. 2020 Oct 19;10.

[51] Lughezzani G, Sun M, Jeldres C, Alasker A, Budäus L, Shariat SF, et al. Adenocarcinoma Versus Urothelial Carcinoma of the Urinary Bladder: Comparison Between Pathologic Stage at Radical Cystectomy and Cancer-specific Mortality. Urology. 2010 Feb;75(2):376-81.

[52] Zaghloul MS, Nouh A, Nazmy M, Ramzy S, Zaghloul AS, Sedira MA, et al. Long-term results of primary adenocarcinoma of the urinary bladder: A report on 192 patients. Urologic Oncology: Seminars and Original Investigations. 2006 Jan;24(1):13-20.

[53] Dutta R, Abdelhalim A, Martin JW, Vernez SL, Faltas B, Lotan Y, et al. Effect of tumor location on survival in urinary bladder adenocarcinoma: A population-based analysis. Urologic Oncology: Seminars and Original Investigations. 2016 Dec 1;34(12):531.e1-531.e6.

[54] Wright JL, Porter MP, Li CI, Lange PH, Lin DW. Differences in survival among patients with urachal and nonurachal adenocarcinomas of the bladder. Cancer. 2006 Aug 15;107(4):721-8.

[55] Edward C, Blomjous M, Vos W, de Voogt HJ, van der Valk P, Meijer CJLM. Small Cell Carcinoma of the Urinary Bladder. 1989.

[56] Berg S, D'Andrea D, Vetterlein MW, Cole AP, Fletcher SA, Krimphove MJ, et al. Impact of adjuvant chemotherapy in patients with adverse features and variant histology at radical cystectomy for muscle-invasive carcinoma of the bladder: Does histologic subtype matter? Cancer. 2019 May 1;125(9):1449-58.

[57] Mukesh M, Cook N, Hollingdale AE, Ainsworth NL, Russell SG. Small cell carcinoma of the urinary bladder: A 15-year retrospective review of treatment and survival in the Anglian Cancer Network. BJU International. 2009 Mar;103(6):747-52.

[58] Vetterlein MW, Mullane S, Seisen T, Lander R, Löppenberg B, Choueiri TK, et al. MP34-11 NEOADJUVANT CHEMOTHERAPY PRIOR TO RADICAL CYSTECTOMY FOR MUSCLE-INVASIVE BLADDER CANCER WITH VARIANT HISTOLOGY. Journal of Urology. 2017 Apr;197(4S).

[59] Wang G, Xiao L, Zhang M, Kamat AM, Siefker-Radtke A, Dinney CP, et al. Small cell carcinoma of the urinary bladder: a clinicopathological and immunohistochemical analysis of 81 cases. Human Pathology. 2018 Sep 1;79:57-65.

[60] Wu Y, Enting D, Rudman S, Chowdhury S. Immunotherapy for urothelial cancer: From BCG to checkpoint inhibitors and beyond. Vol. 15, Expert Review of Anticancer Therapy. Expert Reviews Ltd.; 2015. p. 509-23.

Chapter 3

Gender Disparities in Bladder Cancer

Yingsheng Zhang, Dan Theodorescu and Xue Li

Abstract

Biological sex is an independent risk factor of cancer. Men are three to five times more likely than women to develop bladder cancer even when known risk factors are taken into consideration. Development of sex in mammals is often viewed as a two-step process. The first step is sex determination, of which the XX and XY sex chromosome complements trigger gonad differentiation to form the ovary and testis, respectively. After that, sex hormones secreted by gonads initiate sexually dimorphic differentiation of nongonadal tissues. However, this model has been challenged by recent findings revealing an independent contribution of sex chromosomes to sexual dimorphism. In this chapter, we discuss how the sex chromosomes and sex hormones together cause gender disparities in bladder cancer. We propose a concept of epigenetic sex – epigenetic differences between males and females – and suggest that the sex epigenome is a previously unknown biasing factor contributing to gender disparities in bladder cancer.

Keywords: Bladder Cancer, Gender Disparities, Sex Hormones, Sex Chromosomes, Sex Epigenome, KDM6A, PRC2, COMPASS

1. Introduction

Bladder cancer (BC) originates primarily from the urothelium – the inner lining of bladder lumen. Men are disproportionally affected by the disease. Males are 3–5 times more likely than females to BC [1]. This difference persists even after adjusting other known risk factors [2–5], suggesting that male sex is an independent risk factor of BC.

Typical males have one copy each of the X and Y chromosomes (XY) while females have two copies of the X chromosome (XX). For XY individuals, sex-determining region Y (SRY) gene on the Y chromosome triggers gonadal differentiation to form testes, which secrete androgens and promote male primary and secondary sex characteristics. Females with XX chromosome complement have ovarian development and estrogen secretion leading to female primary and secondary sex characteristics [6].

Strong evidence exists that androgens acting through androgen receptor, promote bladder tumorigenesis [7]. Female gonadal hormones acting through estrogen receptors also influence BC risk albeit playing a minor role when compared to androgens [8]. While sex hormones clearly play important roles in gender disparities in BC, potential role of the sex chromosomes is not nearly as apparent. Because the sex chromosomes (*i.e.,* XX vs. XY) are coupled with the gonadal hormones (*e.g.,* estrogens vs. androgens), it is exceedingly difficult to ascertain independent effects of the sex chromosomes or the gonadal hormones [6]. Creative tools are needed to overcome the challenges of studying sex differences in physiology and disease [9]. Here, we review how the sex hormones and chromosomes function together to cause gender disparities in BC and, furthermore, propose a novel concept of epigenome sex.

2. The impact of biological sex on bladder cancer development

2.1 The role of androgen

A retrospective study revealed that male patients who received α-reductase inhibitors before the diagnosis of BC had better survival and was positively correlated with duration of administration [10]. Similarly, prostate cancer patients who received androgen deprivation therapy (ADT) had a lower incidence of BC compared with patients that did not [11]. Paradoxically, a majority of expression analyses of androgen receptor (AR) in BC patients showed a negative correlation between AR expression and the aggressiveness of BC [12–17]. Offering a possible explanation underlying this observation is our finding that reduced AR expression may lead to upregulation of cancer stem cell related genes such as CD44 [18]. Clearly the role of androgens and AR in BC is complex and likely in molecular and cellular context-dependent manner.

Animal models of BC support the role of androgens/AR in modulating bladder tumorigenesis. Male mice were much more vulnerable than female mice to BC induced by N-butyl-N-(4- hydroxybutyl) nitrosamine (BBN), a bladder-specific carcinogen [19]. This sex difference was blunted by castration. Similarly, Okajima and colleagues have observed male-biased responses to BBN-induced BC in rats. Moreover, administration of Diethylstilbestrol (DES), a nonsteroidal estrogen, suppressed bladder carcinogenesis in male rats. In contrast, testosterone supplementation increased the incidence of BC in female rats [20]. Miyamoto *et al.* have also found that AR knockout (KO) mice, both males and females, were completely protected from BBN-induced BC [21]. Intriguingly, 25% AR KO male mice supplemented with dihydrotestosterone (DHT) had BC after BBN treatment, and 50% of castrated male mice still developed into BC [21]. These data suggest that androgens have AR-independent function in promoting BBN-induced BC, and AR may also function in an androgen-independent manner. In addition, they showed that androgen deprivation or androgen/AR disruption blunted growth of AR-positive human BC cells both *in vitro* and *in vivo* [21]. The genetic evidence of oncogenic role of androgen/AR signaling in bladder carcinogenesis was further confirmed in the subsequent studies. Hsu and colleagues revealed that urothelium-specific conditional KO of AR reduced the risk of BBN-induced BC in male mice. They further showed that AR expression was inversely associated with the level of p53-PCNA-DNA damage pathway, implicating a possible downstream event of AR oncogenic signaling [22]. Johnson *et al.* showed that conditional overexpression of human AR in mouse urothelium was sufficient to promote BBN-induced BC in both sexes and the phenotype in males could be alleviated by castration [23]. Surprisingly, the study also suggested that AR did not function through known molecular pathways which have been previously implicated, including *p53* [22], *Wnt/β-catenin* [24, 25], and *CD24* [26–28]. Therefore, much more work is needed to define the precise role of AR in bladder tumorigenesis.

2.2 The role of estrogens and their receptors

Postmenopausal women had a higher risk of BC and early menopause enhanced this risk, suggesting that female sex hormones protect women from BC development [29–31]. Classical estrogen receptors (ERs) include estrogen receptor α (ERα) and estrogen receptor β (ERβ) [32]. Clinically, inconsistent results existed between the expression of ERα and ERβ and the grades and stages of BC patients although more reports supported that expression of ERα favors a better while ERβ is associated with a worse prognosis [14, 32–38]. Experimentally, both whole body ERα KO or urothelium-specific ERα KO increased the incidence of BBN-induced BC in female mice. Disruption of ERα decreased the expression of Inositol polyphosphate-4-phosphatase, type II (INPP4B), resulting in a higher activation of AKT [39]. On the contrary, whole body deletion of ERβ impeded BBN-induced BC in female mice [40]. Moreover, knockdown (KD) of ERβ suppressed transformation of normal bladder cells and growth of BC cells partly through reducing expression of mini-chromosome maintenance complex component 5 (MCM5) because reintroduction of MCM5 into BC cells blunted ERβ KD phenotype [40]. Interestingly, tamoxifen treatment conferred a chemoprevention in female mice against BBN-induced BC [41]. Since tamoxifen is a selective estrogen-receptor modulator with mixed estrogenic and antiestrogenic activity depending on targeted tissues, it would be interesting to see which ERs, ERα or ERβ, is activated or inhibited and whether any of these receptors plays a more dominant role in the BBN-induced bladder carcinogenesis.

2.3 The role of sex chromosomes in driving gender disparities

A potential role of the sex chromosomes in gender disparities in BC was implicated initially by cancer epidemiological findings of Turner and Klinefelter patients. Turner syndrome is a genetic disorder of female X0 patients who lost one copy of the X chromosome. Conversely, Klinefelter syndrome has two or more copies of the X chromosome among the affected male patients. Turner patients displayed an increased risk of BC [42]; and Klinefelter patients had an overall reduced rate of solid tumors [43]. These observations suggest that an extra copy of X chromosome is tightly associated with low BC risk in both sexes. However, because the sex chromosomes are tightly coupled with their respective sex/gonadal hormones, the confounding effect of sex chromosomes cannot be excluded. As a result, the sex hormone–independent roles of the sex chromosomes have largely been overlooked.

To overcome the aforementioned challenges of studying independent roles of the sex-biasing factors, De Vries *et al.* developed "four-core genotype (FCG)" mouse model to uncouple the link between the sex chromosomes and their corresponding gonadal types [44]. In this model, *Sry* gene is "transferred" from the Y chromosome to an autosome. As a result, the FCG mouse model has four instead of two sex types: 1. XY male with testes (XYM); 2. XX male with testes (XXM); 3. XX female with ovaries (XXF); and 4. XY female with ovaries (XYF). Independent effects of the sex hormones can be evaluated by comparing XXF and XXM mice or XYM and XXM mice without the confounding issue of the sex/gonadal hormones [45]. Similarly, in the comparisons of XXF vs. XYF or XYM vs. XFM, one can evaluate independent effects of the sex chromosomes.

By taking advantage of the FCG mice, we showed that, independent of the sex hormones, the sex chromosomes had a sex-biasing effect on BC development [46]. We further showed that regardless of gonadal sex XY mice had 2.55 times of higher chance of developing BBN-induced BC than XX mice, demonstrating an independent role of the sex chromosomes. This study has also confirmed the sex-biasing role of androgens and further revealed that having testes was 4.71 times more likely than having ovaries to develop BC. More strikingly, wild type male mice with the XY chromosome complement and testes were 12.39 times more likely than wild type female mice with the XX chromosome complement and ovaries. This is unexpected because it is close to the product of 2.55 and 4.71 instead of the sum. Such finding suggests that both the sex chromosomes and the sex hormones have independent and dependent sex-biasing effects on BC. Moreover, the sex chromosomes interact with the sex hormones to amplify the difference (**Figure 1**). The underlying mechanism of interaction between these sex-biasing factors is yet to be defined.

Because the Y chromosome is frequently lost in BC cells and its loss has been associated with a higher cancer risk [47–49], it is less likely that the Y chromosome explains the male dominance in BC. A more reasonable possibility is that copy number difference of the X chromosome may render females better protected than males. To understand the potential tumor suppressing role of the X chromosome, we have examined the X chromosome-linked genes that escape X chromosome inactivation (XCI) (**Figure 1a**) [50], hence, genes that are expressed in higher levels in XX than in XY urothelial cells. By comparing gene expression levels in the bladder urothelium of FCG mice, we have identified Lysine Demethylase 6A (KDM6A)

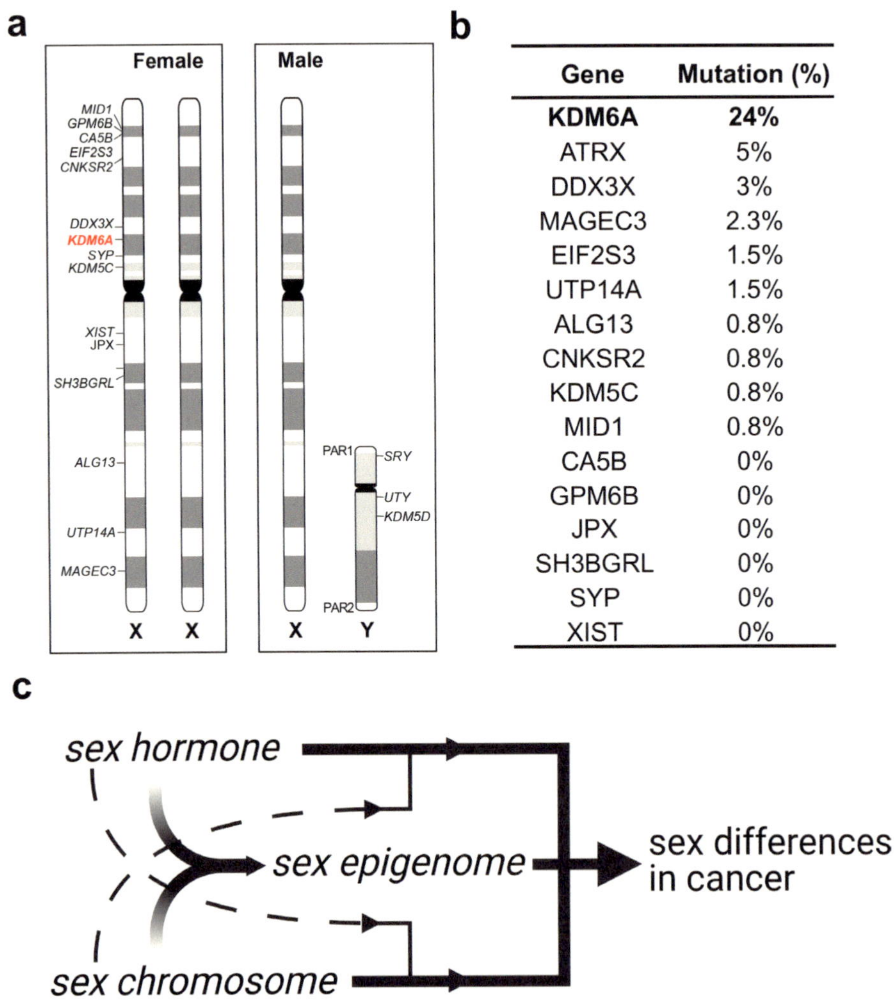

Figure 1.
Major contributing factors of sex differences in bladder cancer. a) Schematic diagram of human sex chromosome complement of XX females and XY males. Genes that are reportedly escaped X-chromosome inactivation (XCI) in both mouse and human are indicated. PAR, Pseudo Autosomal Regions. b) Somatic DNA mutation rate of the candidate XCI escapees in bladder cancer. c) A proposed model that interactions among the sex chromosomes, sex hormones, and sex epigenome amplify male and female differences in bladder cancer.

as a top candidate of X-linked tumor suppressors [46]. *KDM6A* encodes a histone demethylase to remove methyl group from methylated histone H3 at lysine K27 to allow gene transcription. Somatic loss-of-function mutations of human *KDM6A* are tightly associated with BC, suggesting a tumor suppressive function in humans [51–54]. Interestingly, *KDM6A* mutations have been shown to be more common in female patients with non-muscle invasive BC (NMIBC) [54]. We showed that after conditional *Kdm6a* KO in the urothelium of female mice, susceptibility to BBN-induced BC was significantly increased. Similarly, down-regulation or mutation of *KDM6A* was tightly linked to advanced disease stages and poor outcomes among female but not male BC patients [46]. Urothelium-specific *Kdm6a* KO did not exhibit apparent phenotype in male mice. A lack of phenotype in males is potentially due to the compensatory effect of a paralog gene *UTY* on the Y chromosome, albeit that UTY lacks any detectable demethylase activity *in vivo* [55–58]. In addition to *KDM6A,* other X-linked genes have also been suggested to contribute to sex differences in cancer [59]. While these candidate genes were expressed in higher levels in females than in males, their expression was not associated with disease outcomes of BC (**Figure 1b**) [46]. Collectively, these findings suggest that *KDM6A* is a prototypical sex-biasing tumor suppressor in BC.

2.4 The sex epigenome

Through the intrinsic histone demethylase activity, KDM6A regulates downstream gene transcription by antagonizing Polycomb Repressive Complex 2 (PRC2)-dependent epigenetic gene silencing program [60–63]. Specifically, KDM6A catalyzes removal of the methyl groups from histone H3 lysine 27 trimethylation (H3K27me3), making H3K27 available for acetylation (H3K27ac). H3K27me3 and H3K27ac are closely associated with transcription repression and activation, respectively. In a demethylase-independent manner, KDM6A functions in the COMPASS-like protein complex that harbors MLL3/KMT2C and MLL4/KMT2D lysine methyltransferases [64]. KMT2C and KMT2D catalyze formation of H3K4 monomethylation (H3K4me1), which is tightly linked to active transcription enhancers [65–67]. COMPASS and PRC2 display an antagonistic relationship in regulating downstream gene expression [68, 69]. Therefore, *KDM6A* plays a central role in shaping the epigenetic landscape by modulating the PRC2-dependent gene silencing and the COMPASS-dependent gene activation. Nearly 74% of NMIBC and 23% MIBC patients have mutations in *KDM6A* [51, 54]. About 18% and 28% of human BC patients have somatic mutations in *KMT2C* and *KMT2D*, respectively [51]. The sex-biased expression of *KDM6A* suggests that there is an epigenetic difference in bladder urothelium between sexes, hence the sex epigenome. It is conceivable that *KDM6A* plays a critical role in creating an epigenetic barrier to prevent malignant transformation. Females with more *KDM6A* may have a tougher barrier than males to overcome, thereby are less likely to develop BC.

Whole-genome transcriptome analysis of *Kdm6a* knockout urothelium indicates that the p53 tumor suppressor pathway is among the top affected pathways [46]. The canonical p53 downstream gene targets, *Cdkn1a* and *Perp*, which induce cell cycle arrest and apoptosis, respectively, are down-regulated significantly in *KDM6A* knockouts. UM-UC-13, a human BC cell line, lacks functional *KDM6A* due to genomic mutation [70]. Expression of wild type *KDM6A* induces both *CDKN1A* and *PERP* in UM-UC-13 cells while expression of the catalytically-dead form of *KDM6A* only induces *PERP* but not *CDKN1A*, suggesting that *KDM6A* regulates *PERP* gene expression in a demethylase-independent manner. While persistent expression of the enzymatically-dead form of KDM6A is required to suppress UM-UC-13 cell proliferation, a transient expression of *KDM6A* is sufficient to achieve the same result, implying that the demethylase activity of KDM6A results in a lasting protective activity or an epigenetic memory of tumor suppression [46]. In supporting this notion, *Ler et al.* revealed that *KDM6A* mutant BC cells are more vulnerable to the pharmacological inhibition of PRC2 [52]. While the precise mechanism of *KDM6A*-dependent tumor suppression remains to be fully elucidated, we suspect that systematic profiling of the sex epigenome would shed new light on the gender disparities in BC (**Figure 1c**).

3. Conclusion

A new concept of sex epigenome begins to emerge. In addition to gonadal hormones, the copy number difference of the X chromosome between males and females contributes to sex differences in BC - an extra copy of the X chromosome confers a better protection of females. Moreover, there is a cooperative interaction between the sex hormones and chromosomes during BC development. The tumor suppressing effect of the X chromosome is largely mediated by *KDM6A*-dependent epigenetic program, or the sex epigenome. The sex chromosome, sex chromosome, and sex epigenome collectively contribute to sex differences in BC.

Acknowledgements

This work was supported by the NIH/National Cancer Institute (1R01DK110477, 1R01HL136921, and 5R21CA249701 to X.L.).

Conflict of interest

The authors declare no conflict of interest.

Notes/thanks/other declarations

We thank BioRender (https://biorender.com/) for providing the platform for plotting the **Figure 1c**.

Author details

Yingsheng Zhang[1,2], Dan Theodorescu[2,3] and Xue Li[1,2]*

1 Department of Medicine, Cedars-Sinai Samuel Oschin Comprehensive Cancer Institute, Cedars-Sinai Medical Center, Los Angeles, CA, USA

2 Department of Biological Sciences, Cedars-Sinai Samuel Oschin Comprehensive Cancer Institute, Cedars-Sinai Medical Center, Los Angeles, CA, USA

3 Department of Surgery, Cedars-Sinai Samuel Oschin Comprehensive Cancer Institute, Cedars-Sinai Medical Center, Los Angeles, CA, USA

*Address all correspondence to: sean.li@cshc.org

References

[1] Cumberbatch MGK, Jubber I, Black PC, Esperto F, Figueroa JD, Kamat AM, et al. Epidemiology of Bladder Cancer: A Systematic Review and Contemporary Update of Risk Factors in 2018. Vol. 74, European Urology. Elsevier B.V.; 2018. p. 784-95.

[2] Hartge P, Harvey EB, Linehan WM, Silverman DT, Sullivan JW, Hoover RN, et al. Unexplained Excess Risk of Bladder Cancer in Men. JNCI J Natl Cancer Inst [Internet]. 1990 Oct 17 [cited 2021 Mar 9];82(20):1636-40. Available from: https://academic.oup.com/jnci/article-lookup/doi/10.1093/jnci/82.20.1636

[3] Hemelt M, Yamamoto H, Cheng KK, Zeegers MPA. The effect of smoking on the male excess of bladder cancer: A meta-analysis and geographical analyses. Int J Cancer [Internet]. 2009 Jan 15 [cited 2021 Mar 9];124(2):412-9. Available from: http://doi.wiley.com/10.1002/ijc.23856

[4] Krabbe LM, Svatek RS, Shariat SF, Messing E, Lotan Y. Bladder cancer risk: Use of the PLCO and NLST to identify a suitable screening cohort. Urol Oncol Semin Orig Investig. 2015 Feb 1;33(2):65.e19-65.e25.

[5] Siegel RL, Miller KD, Jemal A. Cancer statistics, 2020. CA Cancer J Clin [Internet]. 2020 Jan 8 [cited 2021 Mar 9];70(1):7-30. Available from: https://onlinelibrary.wiley.com/doi/abs/10.3322/caac.21590

[6] Arnold AP. A general theory of sexual differentiation. J Neurosci Res [Internet]. 2017 Jan 2 [cited 2021 Mar 9];95(1-2):291-300. Available from: http://doi.wiley.com/10.1002/jnr.23884

[7] Li P, Chen J, Miyamoto H. Androgen Receptor Signaling in Bladder Cancer. Cancers (Basel) [Internet]. 2017 Feb 22 [cited 2021 Mar 19];9(12):20. Available from: http://www.mdpi.com/2072-6694/9/2/20

[8] Hsu NR| U. Role of oestrogen receptors in bladder cancer development. Nat Publ Gr [Internet]. 2013 [cited 2021 Mar 19];10:317-26. Available from: www.nature.com/nrurol

[9] Arnold AP. Conceptual frameworks and mouse models for studying sex differences in physiology and disease: Why compensation changes the game [Internet]. Vol. 259, Experimental Neurology. Academic Press Inc.; 2014 [cited 2021 Mar 28]. p. 2-9. Available from: /pmc/articles/PMC4125548/

[10] Mäkelä VJ, Kotsar A, Tammela TLJ, Murtola TJ. Bladder Cancer Survival of Men Receiving 5α-Reductase Inhibitors. J Urol. 2018 Oct 1;200(4):743-8.

[11] Izumi K, Taguri M, Miyamoto H, Hara Y, Kishida T, Chiba K, et al. Androgen deprivation therapy prevents bladder cancer recurrence. Oncotarget [Internet]. 2014 [cited 2021 Mar 11];5(24):12665-74. Available from: /pmc/articles/PMC4350350/

[12] Laor E, Schiffman ZJ, Braunstein JD, Reid RE, Tolia BM, Koss LG, et al. Androgen receptors in bladder tumors. Urology. 1985 Feb 1;25(2):161-3.

[13] Miyamoto H, Yao JL, Chaux A, Zheng Y, Hsu I, Izumi K, et al. Expression of androgen and oestrogen receptors and its prognostic significance in urothelial neoplasm of the urinary bladder. BJU Int [Internet]. 2012 Jun 1 [cited 2021 Mar 10];109(11):1716-26. Available from: http://doi.wiley.com/10.1111/j.1464-410X.2011.10706.x

[14] Tuygun C, Kankaya D, Imamoglu A, Sertcelik A, Zengin K, Oktay M, et al. Sex-specific hormone receptors in urothelial carcinomas of the human urinary bladder: A comparative analysis

of clinicopathological features and survival outcomes according to receptor expression. Urol Oncol Semin Orig Investig. 2011 Jan 1;29(1):43-51.

[15] Nam JK, Park SW, Lee SD, Chung MK. Prognostic Value of Sex-Hormone Receptor Expression in Non-Muscle-Invasive Bladder Cancer. Yonsei Med J [Internet]. 2014 Sep 1 [cited 2021 Mar 10];55(5):1214. Available from: https://eymj.org/DOIx.php?id=10.3349/ymj.2014.55.5.1214

[16] Williams EM, Higgins JP, Ankur ·, Sangoi R, Mckenney JK, Troxell ML. Androgen receptor immunohistochemistry in genitourinary neoplasms. Int Urol Nephrol. 2015;3:81-5.

[17] Boorjian S, Ugras S, Mongan NP, Gudas LJ, You X, Tickoo SK, et al. Androgen receptor expression is inversely correlated with pathologic tumor stage in bladder cancer. Urology. 2004 Aug 1;64(2):383-8.

[18] Sottnik JL, Vanderlinden LA, Joshi M, Chauca-Diaz A, Owens C, Hansel DE, et al. Androgen Receptor Regulates CD44 Expression in Bladder Cancer. Cancer Res [Internet]. 2021 Mar 9 [cited 2021 Mar 26];canres.3095.2020. Available from: http://cancerres.aacrjournals.org/lookup/doi/10.1158/0008-5472.CAN-20-3095

[19] Bertram JS, Craig AW. Specific induction of bladder cancer in mice by butyl-(4-hydroxybutyl)-nitrosamine and the effects of hormonal modifications on the sex difference in response. Eur J Cancer. 1972 Dec 1;8(6):587-94.

[20] Okajima E, Hiramatsu T, Iriya K, Ijuin M, Matsushima S, Yamada K. Effect of sex hormones on development of urinary bladder tumours in rats induced by N-butyl-N-(4-hydroxybutyl) nitrosamine. Urol Res [Internet]. 1975 Aug [cited 2021 Mar 10];3(2):73-9. Available from: https://link.springer.com/article/10.1007/BF00256185

[21] Miyamoto H, Yang Z, Chen Y-T, Ishiguro H, Uemura H, Kubota Y, et al. Promotion of Bladder Cancer Development and Progression by Androgen Receptor Signals. JNCI J Natl Cancer Inst [Internet]. 2007 Apr 4 [cited 2021 Mar 10];99(7):558-68. Available from: https://academic.oup.com/jnci/article-lookup/doi/10.1093/jnci/djk113

[22] Hsu JW, Hsu I, Xu D, Miyamoto H, Liang L, Wu XR, et al. Decreased tumorigenesis and mortality from bladder cancer in mice lacking urothelial androgen receptor. Am J Pathol. 2013 May 1;182(5):1811-20.

[23] Johnson DT, Hooker E, Luong R, Yu E-J, He Y, Gonzalgo ML, et al. Conditional Expression of the Androgen Receptor Increases Susceptibility of Bladder Cancer in Mice. Agoulnik IU, editor. PLoS One [Internet]. 2016 Feb 10 [cited 2021 Mar 10];11(2):e0148851. Available from: https://dx.plos.org/10.1371/journal.pone.0148851

[24] Lin C, Yin Y, Stemler K, Humphrey P, Kibel AS, Mysorekar IU, et al. Constitutive β-catenin activation induces male-specific tumorigenesis in the bladder urothelium. Cancer Res [Internet]. 2013 Oct 1 [cited 2021 Mar 21];73(19):5914-25. Available from: http://cancerres.aacrjournals.org/

[25] Li Y, Zheng Y, Izumi K, Ishiguro H, Ye B, Li F, et al. Androgen activates β-catenin signaling in bladder cancer cells. Endocr Relat Cancer [Internet]. 2013 Jun 20 [cited 2021 Mar 21];20(3):293-304. Available from: https://erc.bioscientifica.com/view/journals/erc/20/3/293.xml

[26] Thomas S, Harding MA, Smith SC, Overdevest JB, Nitz MD, Frierson HF, et al. CD24 is an effector of HIF-1-driven primary tumor growth and metastasis.

Cancer Res [Internet]. 2012 Nov 1 [cited 2021 Mar 21];72(21):5600-12. Available from: http://cancerres.aacrjournals.org/

[27] Overdevest JB, Thomas S, Kristiansen G, Hansel DE, Smith SC, Theodorescu D. CD24 offers a therapeutic target for control of bladder cancer metastasis based on a requirement for lung colonization. Cancer Res [Internet]. 2011 Jun 1 [cited 2021 Mar 21];71(11):3802-11. Available from: http://cancerres.aacrjournals.org/

[28] Overdevest JB, Knubel KH, Duex JE, Thomas S, Nitz MD, Harding MA, et al. CD24 expression is important in male urothelial tumorigenesis and metastasis in mice and is androgen regulated. Proc Natl Acad Sci U S A [Internet]. 2012 Dec 18 [cited 2021 Mar 21];109(51):E3588-96. Available from: www.pnas.org/cgi/doi/10.1073/pnas.1113960109

[29] McGrath M, Michaud DS, De Vivo I. Hormonal and Reproductive Factors and the Risk of Bladder Cancer in Women. Am J Epidemiol [Internet]. 2006 Feb 1 [cited 2021 Mar 10];163(3):236-44. Available from: http://academic.oup.com/aje/article/163/3/236/59618/Hormonal-and-Reproductive-Factors-and-the-Risk-of

[30] Dietrich K, Demidenko E, Schned A, Zens MS, Heaney J, Karagas MR. Parity, early menopause and the incidence of bladder cancer in women: A case-control study and meta-analysis. Eur J Cancer. 2011 Mar 1;47(4):592-9.

[31] Wolpert BJ, Amr S, Ezzat S, Saleh D, Gouda I, Loay I, et al. Estrogen exposure and bladder cancer risk in Egyptian women. Maturitas. 2010 Dec 1;67(4):353-7.

[32] Teng J, Wang ZY, Jarrard DF, Bjorling DE. Roles of estrogen receptor α and β in modulating urothelial cell proliferation. Endocr Relat Cancer [Internet]. 2008 Mar [cited 2021 Mar 11];15(1):351-64. Available from: /pmc/articles/PMC3513362/

[33] Basakci A, Kirkali Z, Tuzel E, Yorukoglu K, Mungan MU, Sade M. Prognostic significance of estrogen receptor expression in superficial transitional cell carcinoma of the urinary bladder. Eur Urol. 2002 Mar 1;41(3):342-5.

[34] Shen SS, Smith CL, Hsieh J-T, Yu J, Kim IY, Jian W, et al. Expression of estrogen receptors-α and -β in bladder cancer cell lines and human bladder tumor tissue. Cancer [Internet]. 2006 Jun 15 [cited 2021 Mar 11];106(12):2610-6. Available from: http://doi.wiley.com/10.1002/cncr.21945

[35] Miyamoto H, Yao JL, Chaux A, Zheng Y, Hsu I, Izumi K, et al. Expression of androgen and oestrogen receptors and its prognostic significance in urothelial neoplasm of the urinary bladder. BJU Int [Internet]. 2012 Jun 1 [cited 2021 Mar 11];109(11):1716-26. Available from: http://doi.wiley.com/10.1111/j.1464-410X.2011.10706.x

[36] Bolenz C, Lotan Y, Ashfaq R, Shariat SF. Estrogen and Progesterone Hormonal Receptor Expression in Urothelial Carcinoma of the Bladder. Eur Urol [Internet]. 2009 Dec 7 [cited 2021 Mar 11];56(6):1093-5. Available from: https://linkinghub.elsevier.com/retrieve/pii/S0302283809006769

[37] Croft PR, Lathrop SL, Feddersen RM, Joste NE. Estrogen receptor expression in papillary urothelial carcinoma of the bladder and ovarian transitional cell carcinoma. In: Archives of Pathology and Laboratory Medicine [Internet]. Arch Pathol Lab Med; 2005 [cited 2021 Mar 11]. p. 194-9. Available from: https://pubmed.ncbi.nlm.nih.gov/15679420/

[38] Kontos S, Kominea A, Melachrinou M, Balampani E,

Sotiropoulou-Bonikou G. Inverse expression of estrogen receptor-β and nuclear factor-κB in urinary bladder carcinogenesis. Int J Urol [Internet]. 2010 Sep 1 [cited 2021 Mar 11];17(9):801-9. Available from: http://doi.wiley.com/10.1111/j.1442-2042.2010.02603.x

[39] Hsu I, Yeh CR, Slavin S, Miyamoto H, Netto GJ, Tsai YC, et al. Estrogen receptor alpha prevents bladder cancer development via INPP4B inhibited Akt pathway in vitro and in vivo. Oncotarget [Internet]. 2014 [cited 2021 Mar 11];5(17):7917-35. Available from: /pmc/articles/PMC4202170/

[40] Hsu I, Chuang K-L, Slavin S, Da J, Lim W-X, Pang S-T, et al. Suppression of ERβ signaling via ERβ knockout or antagonist protects against bladder cancer development. Carcinogenesis [Internet]. 2014 Mar 1 [cited 2021 Mar 11];35(3):651-61. Available from: https://academic.oup.com/carcin/article-lookup/doi/10.1093/carcin/bgt348

[41] George SK, Tovar-Sepulveda V, Shen SS, Jian W, Zhang Y, Hilsenbeck SG, et al. Chemoprevention of BBN-induced bladder carcinogenesis by the selective Estrogen receptor modulator tamoxifen. Transl Oncol. 2013 Jun 1;6(3):244-55.

[42] Schoemaker MJ, Swerdlow AJ, Higgins CD, Wright AF, Jacobs PA. Cancer incidence in women with Turner syndrome in Great Britain: a national cohort study. Lancet Oncol [Internet]. 2008 Mar [cited 2021 Mar 11];9(3):239-46. Available from: https://pubmed.ncbi.nlm.nih.gov/18282803/

[43] Ji J, Zöller B, Sundquist J, Sundquist K. Risk of solid tumors and hematological malignancy in persons with Turner and Klinefelter syndromes: A national cohort study. Int J Cancer [Internet]. 2016 Aug 15 [cited 2021 Mar 11];139(4):754-8. Available from: http://doi.wiley.com/10.1002/ijc.30126

[44] De Vries GJ, Rissman EF, Simerly RB, Yang LY, Scordalakes EM, Auger CJ, et al. A model system for study of sex chromosome effects on sexually dimorphic neural and behavioral traits. J Neurosci [Internet]. 2002 Oct 15 [cited 2021 Mar 11];22(20):9005-14. Available from: https://www.jneurosci.org/content/22/20/9005

[45] Burgoyne PS, Arnold AP. A primer on the use of mouse models for identifying direct sex chromosome effects that cause sex differences in non-gonadal tissues [Internet]. Vol. 7, Biology of Sex Differences. BioMed Central Ltd.; 2016 [cited 2021 Mar 22]. p. 1-21. Available from: /pmc/articles/PMC5154145/

[46] Kaneko S, Li X. X chromosome protects against bladder cancer in females via a KDM6A-dependent epigenetic mechanism. Sci Adv [Internet]. 2018 Jun 13 [cited 2021 Mar 10];4(6):eaar5598. Available from: http://advances.sciencemag.org/

[47] Fadl-Elmula I, Gorunova L, Mandahl N, Elfving P, Lundgren R, Mitelman F, et al. Karyotypic characterization of urinary bladder transitional cell carcinomas. Genes Chromosom Cancer [Internet]. 2000 Nov 1 [cited 2021 Mar 11];29(3):256-65. Available from: https://onlinelibrary.wiley.com/doi/full/10.1002/1098-2264%282000%299999%3A9999%3C%3A%3AAID-GCC1034%3E3.0.CO%3B2-O

[48] Minner S, Kilgué A, Stahl P, Weikert S, Rink M, Dahlem R, et al. Y chromosome loss is a frequent early event in urothelial bladder cancer. Pathology. 2010;42(4):356-9.

[49] Forsberg LA, Rasi C, Malmqvist N, Davies H, Pasupulati S, Pakalapati G, et al. Mosaic loss of chromosome y in peripheral blood is associated with shorter survival and higher risk of

cancer. Nat Genet [Internet]. 2014 Apr 28 [cited 2021 Mar 11];46(6):624-8. Available from: https://www.nature.com/articles/ng.2966

[50] Tukiainen T, Villani AC, Yen A, Rivas MA, Marshall JL, Satija R, et al. Landscape of X chromosome inactivation across human tissues. Nature [Internet]. 2017 Oct 11 [cited 2021 Mar 19];550(7675):244-8. Available from: https://www.nature.com/articles/nature24265

[51] Robertson AG, Kim J, Al-Ahmadie H, Bellmunt J, Guo G, Cherniack AD, et al. Comprehensive Molecular Characterization of Muscle-Invasive Bladder Cancer. Cell. 2017 Oct 19;171(3):540-556.e25.

[52] Ler LD, Ghosh S, Chai X, Thike AA, Heng HL, Siew EY, et al. Loss of tumor suppressor KDM6A amplifies PRC2-regulated transcriptional repression in bladder cancer and can be targeted through inhibition of EZH2. Sci Transl Med [Internet]. 2017 Feb 22 [cited 2021 Mar 11];9(378). Available from: http://stm.sciencemag.org/

[53] Nordentoft I, Lamy P, Birkenkamp-Demtröder K, Shumansky K, Vang S, Hornshøj H, et al. Mutational context and diverse clonal development in early and late bladder cancer. Cell Rep. 2014 Jun 12;7(5):1649-63.

[54] Hurst CD, Alder O, Platt FM, Droop A, Stead LF, Burns JE, et al. Genomic Subtypes of Non-invasive Bladder Cancer with Distinct Metabolic Profile and Female Gender Bias in KDM6A Mutation Frequency. Cancer Cell. 2017 Nov 13;32(5):701-715.e7.

[55] Shpargel KB, Sengoku T, Yokoyama S, Magnuson T. UTX and UTY Demonstrate Histone Demethylase-Independent Function in Mouse Embryonic Development. Wysocka J, editor. PLoS Genet [Internet]. 2012 Sep 27 [cited 2021 Mar 11];8(9):e1002964. Available from: https://dx.plos.org/10.1371/journal.pgen.1002964

[56] Wang C, Lee JE, Cho YW, Xiao Y, Jin Q, Liu C, et al. UTX regulates mesoderm differentiation of embryonic stem cells independent of H3K27 demethylase activity. Proc Natl Acad Sci U S A [Internet]. 2012 Sep 18 [cited 2021 Mar 11];109(38):15324-9. Available from: www.pnas.org/cgi/doi/10.1073/pnas.1204166109

[57] Gozdecka M, Meduri E, Mazan M, Tzelepis K, Dudek M, Knights AJ, et al. UTX-mediated enhancer and chromatin remodeling suppresses myeloid leukemogenesis through noncatalytic inverse regulation of ETS and GATA programs. Nat Genet [Internet]. 2018 Jun 1 [cited 2021 Mar 11];50(6):883-94. Available from: https://doi.org/10.1038/s41588-018-0114-z

[58] Welstead GG, Creyghton MP, Bilodeau S, Cheng AW, Markoulaki S, Young RA, et al. X-linked H3K27me3 demethylase Utx is required for embryonic development in a sex-specific manner. Proc Natl Acad Sci U S A [Internet]. 2012 Aug 7 [cited 2021 Mar 11];109(32):13004-9. Available from: www.pnas.org/cgi/doi/10.1073/pnas.1210787109

[59] Dunford A, Weinstock DM, Savova V, Schumacher SE, Cleary JP, Yoda A, et al. Tumor-suppressor genes that escape from X-inactivation contribute to cancer sex bias. Nat Genet [Internet]. 2017 Jan 1 [cited 2021 Mar 21];49(1):10-6. Available from: /pmc/articles/PMC5206905/

[60] Agger K, Cloos PAC, Christensen J, Pasini D, Rose S, Rappsilber J, et al. UTX and JMJD3 are histone H3K27 demethylases involved in HOX gene regulation and development. Nature [Internet]. 2007 Oct 11 [cited 2021 Mar 19];449(7163):731-4. Available from:

https://www.nature.com/articles/nature06145

[61] Hong SH, Cho YW, Yu LR, Yu H, Veenstra TD, Ge K. Identification of JmjC domain-containing UTX and JMJD3 as histone H3 lysine 27 demethylases. Proc Natl Acad Sci U S A [Internet]. 2007 Nov 20 [cited 2021 Mar 22];104(47):18439-44. Available from: www.pnas.orgcgidoi10.1073pnas.0707292104

[62] Lan F, Bayliss PE, Rinn JL, Whetstine JR, Wang JK, Chen S, et al. A histone H3 lysine 27 demethylase regulates animal posterior development. Nature [Internet]. 2007 Oct 11 [cited 2021 Mar 22];449(7163):689-94. Available from: https://www.nature.com/articles/nature06192

[63] Min GL, Villa R, Trojer P, Norman J, Yan KP, Reinberg D, et al. Demethylation of H3K27 regulates polycomb recruitment and H2A ubiquitination. Science (80-) [Internet]. 2007 Oct 19 [cited 2021 Mar 19];318(5849):447-50. Available from: http://science.sciencemag.org/

[64] Cho YW, Hong T, Hong SH, Guo H, Yu H, Kim D, et al. PTIP associates with MLL3- and MLL4-containing histone H3 lysine 4 methyltransferase complex. J Biol Chem. 2007 Jul 13;282(28):20395-406.

[65] Wang SP, Tang Z, Chen CW, Shimada M, Koche RP, Wang LH, et al. A UTX-MLL4-p300 Transcriptional Regulatory Network Coordinately Shapes Active Enhancer Landscapes for Eliciting Transcription. Mol Cell. 2017 Jul 20;67(2):308-321.e6.

[66] Dorighi KM, Swigut T, Henriques T, Bhanu N V., Scruggs BS, Nady N, et al. Mll3 and Mll4 Facilitate Enhancer RNA Synthesis and Transcription from Promoters Independently of H3K4 Monomethylation. Mol Cell. 2017 May 18;66(4):568-576.e4.

[67] Rickels R, Herz H-M, Sze CC, Cao K, Morgan MA, Collings CK, et al. Histone H3K4 monomethylation catalyzed by Trr and mammalian COMPASS-like proteins at enhancers is dispensable for development and viability. Nat Genet Vol. 2017;49(11).

[68] Cenik BK, Shilatifard A. COMPASS and SWI/SNF complexes in development and disease [Internet]. Vol. 22, Nature Reviews Genetics. Nature Research; 2021 [cited 2021 Mar 19]. p. 38-58. Available from: www.nature.com/nrg

[69] Piunti A, Shilatifard A. Epigenetic balance of gene expression by Polycomb and COMPASS families. Science (80-) [Internet]. 2016 Jun 3 [cited 2021 Mar 19];352(6290):aad9780. Available from: https://www.sciencemag.org/lookup/doi/10.1126/science.aad9780

[70] Nickerson ML, Witte N, Im KM, Turan S, Owens C, Misner K, et al. Molecular analysis of urothelial cancer cell lines for modeling tumor biology and drug response. Oncogene [Internet]. 2017 Jan 5 [cited 2021 Mar 22];36(1):35-46. Available from: /pmc/articles/PMC5140783/

Chapter 4

Robot-Assisted Radical Cystectomy with Intra-Corporeal Neo-Bladder

Víctor Enrique Corona-Montes, Eduardo Gonzalez-Cuenca, Laurent López, Juan Eduardo Sánchez-Núñez and Richard Gaston

Abstract

The purpose of this chapter is to provide a step-by-step description of the robot-assisted radical cystectomy with an intra-corporeal neo-bladder technique and a recent review of its outcomes. The procedure is also known as anterior pelvic exenteration or cysto-prostatectomy in the case of female or male respectively. Radical cystectomy (RC) is the gold standard treatment for muscle-invasive bladder cancer, but there are also several surgical indications for non-muscle-invasive bladder cancer. In the past years, minimally invasive surgery and the da Vinci system technology have played a major role in this procedure, with description of brand-new techniques and specific approaches for the creation of a continent urinary reservoir. The following chapter provides a detailed description of the robot-assisted radical cystectomy (RARC) with Y-shaped intra-corporeal bladder as well as a literary review of distinct perioperative, functional and oncological outcomes from the available RARC randomized controlled trials. Despite its high cost and complexity, the intra-corporeal technique has become widely popular around the world and is used more frequently each time. The described data in this chapter, demonstrates that morbidity can be reduced whilst simultaneously offer non-inferior oncological results and less intraoperative blood loss in contrast to the open RC approach.

Keywords: radical cystectomy, neo-bladder, urinary diversion, robotic surgery, bladder cancer

1. Introduction

The Radical Cystectomy with extended pelvic lymph node dissection has evolved dramatically with the emergence of new robotic technological advancements.

Bladder cancer is a broad-spectrum disease, from papillary urothelial non-invasive tumor to aggressive invasive lesions that require radical and multi-modal management [1]. Radical cystectomy (RC) has been the gold standard treatment for muscle-invasive bladder cancer [2, 3].

Historically, in the early 1800s, RC was performed with an open approach however the principles for the current technique were published in 1949 by Marshall and Withmore. Both authors listed some important disadvantages of this procedure such as its high impact on morbidity, overall survival rate and patient's quality of life [4, 5].

Over the years, this procedure has been redefined thanks to the increasing new technology developed around minimally invasive approaches (laparoscopy and robotic-assisted laparoscopy), that implies numerous advantages compared with standard procedures, including decreased blood lost, postoperative narcotic use, time to flatus, time to bowel movement and length of stay [2, 6–9].

Menon and his group developed the robotic-assisted technique and approach to the prostate at the beginning of the 2000s. Based on the rationale that radical prostatectomy could be performed with the robot-assisted approach, this principle was applied to multiple surgeries including radical cystectomy and urinary diversion [10–12].

Initial laparoscopic experience on radical cystectomy was described by two main groups, the first one leaded by Parra et al., who reported their initial experience in the department of Surgery of Saint Louis University School of Medicine in Missouri in 1992 and the second by Sanchez de Badajoz et al., who described several case reports of RC, lymph node dissection and laparoscopic urinary diversion in 1995 in the department of Surgery of the University of Malaga, Spain [4, 12, 13].

First reports of robotic-assisted radical cystectomy (RARC) were reported by Menon and colleagues in Egypt in 2003, where they concluded and published that this approach was both safe and feasible. Recent publications explore the potential to improve morbidity and oncological outcomes [4, 10, 14].

According to the National Inpatient Sample, RARC has gained popularity among urologic surgeons as the preferred minimally invasive approach for bladder malignancies and continues to evolve throughout time. Nowadays, highly experienced surgeons have adventured to perform intra-corporeal urinary diversion reconstruction and have compared general and oncological outcomes as well as health-related quality of life in a large number of patients [4–15].

2. Anatomical landmarks

The bladder is an extra-peritoneal muscular urine reservoir located behind the pubic symphysis in the pelvis. The male bladder consists of a distensible structure, formed at the level of the bladder neck by involuntary internal sphincter fibers. The standard surgical approach of the bladder is through a transperitoneal access. The cul-de-sac separates the rectum and the seminal vesicles from this deep pelvic area. The bladder neck is surrounded by the lateral ligaments and the arch of the pelvic fascia. The anterior portion of the bladder, is supported by the pubo-prostatic ligaments. In the female, the peritoneum lies anterior and superior to the vagina's wall on the Douglas space, anteriorly tendinous arch lateral and pubovesical ligaments.

The bladder is irrigated by the branches of the internal iliac artery:

- Antero-superior baldder: superior vesical artery

- Posterior-inferior bladder: Inferior vesical artery (vaginal artery in the females)

The venous drainage coalesces in a venous plexus and prostatic venous plexus in the male and through the uterus vaginal plexus in the female, which ultimately drains into the internal iliac vein.

The lymphatic system has a supero-lateral drainage to the external iliac lymph nodes, the fundus and neck of the bladder drains to the internal iliac lymph nodes and the sacral lymph nodes [16].

The innervation is provided by presynaptic sympathetic fiber form T11-L2/3 and presynaptic parasympathetic fibers from S2-S4 and postsynaptic neurons in the wall of the bladder [16].

3. Surgical indications for cystectomy

The rationale of performing a cystectomy for malignancy is the outcome and implications of such minimally invasive surgery where continence, potency and sexual function, plus enhanced recovery programs, play a better role. Nowadays, the robotic technique has been further developed by several groups, with more technical variations and anatomical findings, having the sparing of structures as part of the actual benefits. The lymphadenectomy plays also a very important role and their oncological results are quite strong. The **Figure 1** below shows an algorithm of disease management [17, 18].

3.1 Immediate RC to patients with non-muscle-invasive tumors

- T1 tumors (high-risk progression)
- G3 (high grade) tumors.
- CIS.
- Multiple, recurrent and large (> 3 cm) TaG1G2/low-grade tumors.

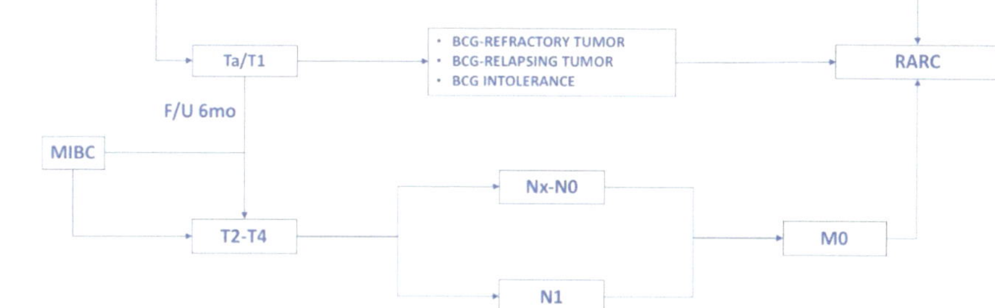

**NMIBC, NON-MUSCLE INVASIVE BLADDER CANCER; MIBC, MUSCLE-INVASIVE BLADDER CANCER, CIS, CARCINOMA IN SITU; BCG, BACILLUS CALMETE-GUERIN; RARC, ROBOTIC-ASSISTED RADICAL CYSTECTOMY; F/U, FOLLOW-UP

Figure 1.
Disease management algorithm.

Subgroup of highest-risk tumors:

- T1G3/high-grade associated with concurrent bladder CIS.
- Multiple and/or large T1G3/high grade and/or recurrent T1G3/high-grade.
- T1G3/high-grade with CIS in the prostatic urethra.
- Some forms of variant histology of UC.
- Lymphovascular invasion.

pTa: for refractory, relapsing or intolerance to BCG treatment.

pT1: multifocality, lamina propia invasion, recurrence after intravesical therapy, CIS.

3.2 RC to patients with muscle-invasive tumors

- pT2-T4.

4. Contraindications for urinary diversion

4.1 Absolute

- Renal function or hepatic function compromised (serum creatinine >2 mg/dl).
- Involvement of the distal urethra to the prostate or involvement of bladder neck.
- Presence of Metastatic disease.
- Physical disability (mental capability and hand dexterity).

4.2 Relative

- Advance age (>70y).
- Radiation to pelvis.
- Bowel disease
- Previous urinary incontinence or damaged rhabdosphincter [17, 18].

5. Surgical technique

5.1 Trocar placements

First robotic port is a 8-mm trocar for the camera, positioned in the midline 2 cm higher to the umbilicus. Robotic port for the scissors is placed in the lateral border of right rectus muscle. Second robotic port for the bipolar forceps in the left lateral border of rectus muscle and the third port for robotic grasp is placed as lateral about 3 fingerbreadths from the anterior-superior iliac spine. One more 5-mm port for suction, clip device and laparoscopic grasp, and a 15-mm port between the camera port and the right robotic one in a triangle position to avoid conflicts, these last port will be use for mechanical staplers. Patient is placed in a steep Trendelenburg position and the robotic system is docked [19].

5.2 Cystectomy and lymph node dissection

5.2.1 Female (anterior pelvic exenteration)

The technique starts with the section of the ovarian ligament following down this step will be also the start of the extended pelvic lymph node dissection reaching a better exposition of the ureter and later the bladder pedicles on the right side (**Figure 2**).

Once the lymph nodes are dissected medial to the ureter it can be visualized from the cross up over the iliac artery bifurcation, the ureter is perfectly identify and clip and transected then the lateral nodes are accomplished avoiding any injury of the hypogastric vessels and the obturator nerve preservation (**Figure 3**).

The common iliac artery bifurcation with-out the nodes shows the internal and external iliac arteries progressively dissected. The operative field view allows the identification of the bladder pedicles which are clipped or transected by ultrasonic device, the left ureter is clip and transected, lateral to this last one we follow the pedicle (**Figure 4**).

The same dissection is reproduced in the left side for the lymph node and the removed nodes are placed in an Endobag. It is then that both ureters are clipped and transected distally. In the case of uterus presence the pedicles are also clip by ultrasonic energy following the hypogastric artery to find the uterus branches. Because previously lymph node dissection and ureteral identification, uterus and vesical pedicles are easier to identify during exposition and dissection. Both pedicles are controlled and the lower plane of the bladder is follow by the anterior vaginal wall in assistance of a vaginal valve (**Figure 5**) [19, 20].

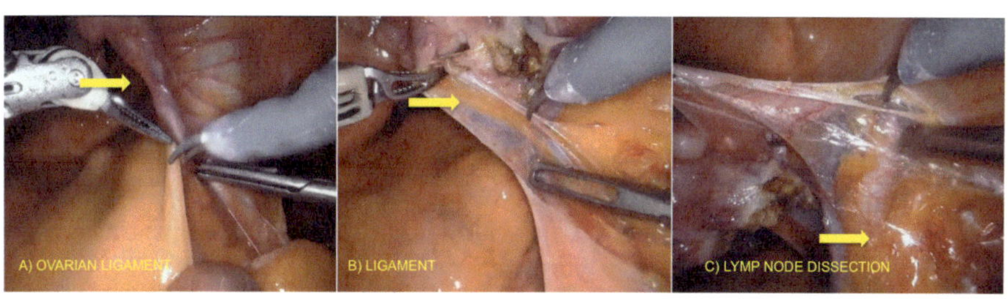

Figure 2.
Female ligament transection and lymph node.

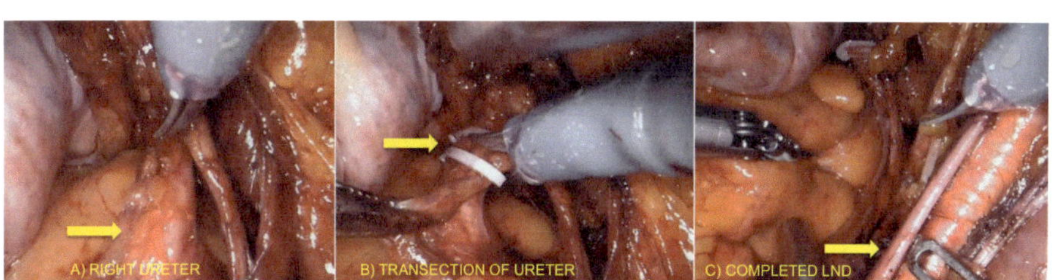

Figure 3.
Right ureter identification and lymphadenectomy.

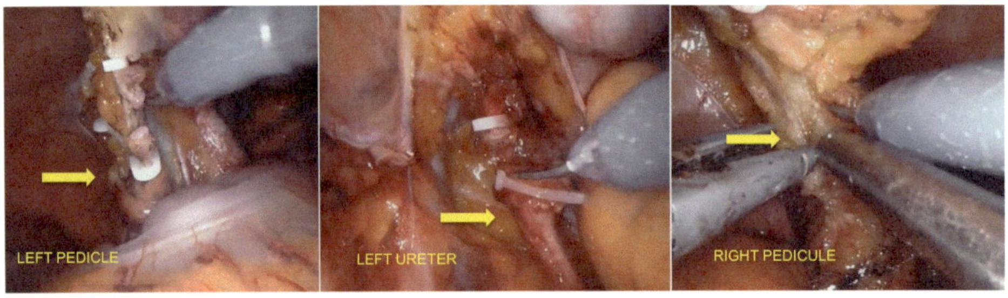

Figure 4.
Left ureter and pedicle identification.

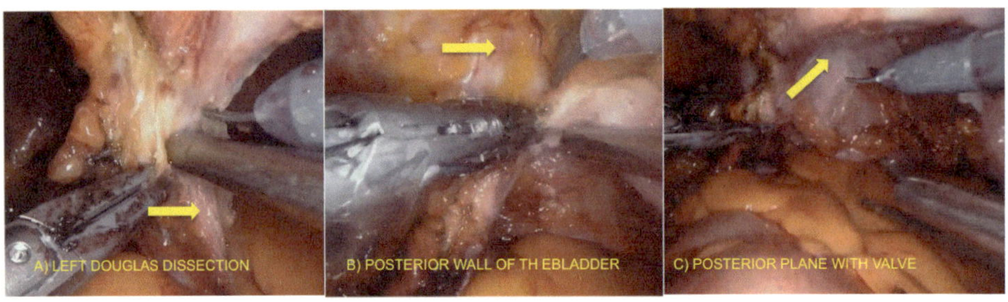

Figure 5.
Anterior wall of the vaginal plane and anterior bladder.

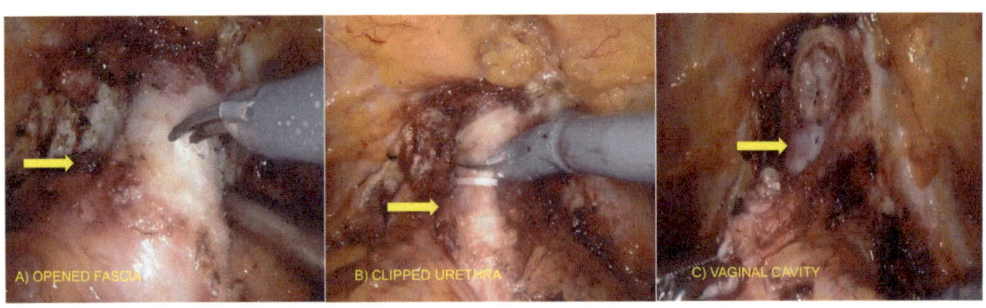

Figure 6.
Urethra dissection and vaginal cavity.

The dissection of the lateral surfaces of the bladder is extended, following the medial umbilical ligaments to the medial plane, the reflection of the endopelvic fascia is visualized and open it, the anterior urethra space is created and the urethra is clipped at the tip and transected safely, the specimen can be retrieval by the vaginal cavity (**Figure 6**) [21].

5.2.2 Male (cysto-prostatectomy)

When performing a lateral approach to the prostate the dissection of the lateral surface of the bladder starts on the right side, down dissection goes proximal to the prostatic pedicle following along the prostatic capsule and the seminal vesicle is identify [19]. The dissection starts lateral to the umbilical ligament, an incision is perform to the peritoneum until the finding of the ureter (**Figure 7**).

Following the ligament and medial will find the right ureter, while dissecting the perineotomy starts a little bit medial but not full open, just to continuo down and to expose the Vas Deferens and the Seminal Vesicle. The ureter is transected and clipped (**Figure 8**).

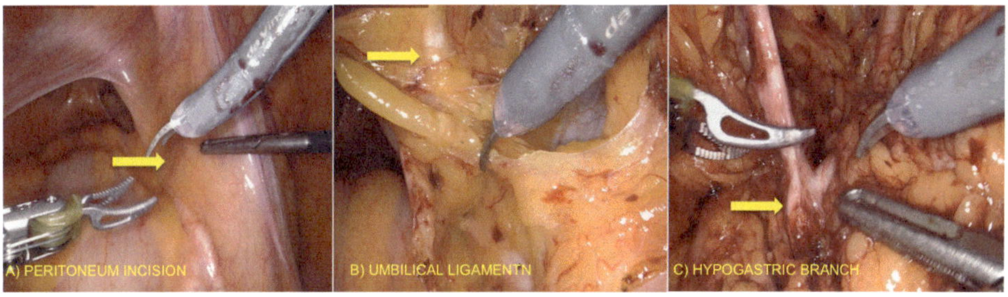

Figure 7.
Peritoneum incision and umbilical identification and transection.

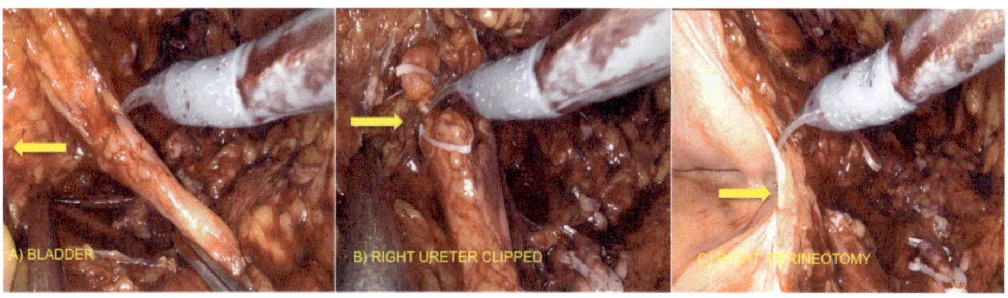

Figure 8.
Right ureter and half perineotomy.

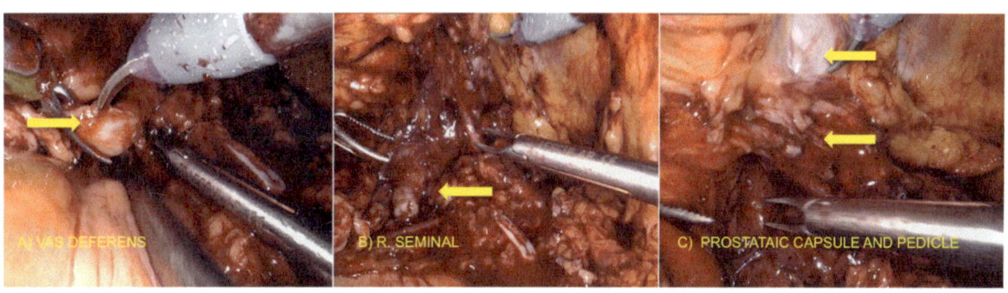

Figure 9.
Right lateral prostatic dissection.

The medial and ventral surfaces of the Seminal vesicle is transect, preserving the middle part and tip avoiding parasympathetic fibers damage in selected cases. The prostate vesicular angle is follow laterally to the apex [20–23] (**Figure 9**).

The same steps are replicated for the left side, starting with incision in the peritoneum lateral to the umbilical ligament, then ureter identification and transection. The lateral pedicles form bladder and prostate are identified and the seminal vesicle and vas are transected. The lateral face of the prostate is follow till the apex, and the Denonvillier's fascia is released (**Figure 10**).

Ligaments and endopelvic fascia are preserved, Santorini plexus is push up without any stich, the urethra is clip transected with the maximum length possible. The specimen is placed in an Endobag (**Figure 11**).

5.3 Neo-bladder creation

The creation of a Y-neobladder intra-corporeal technique following from the Clinique Saint-Augustin is described and showed step by step. The neobladder

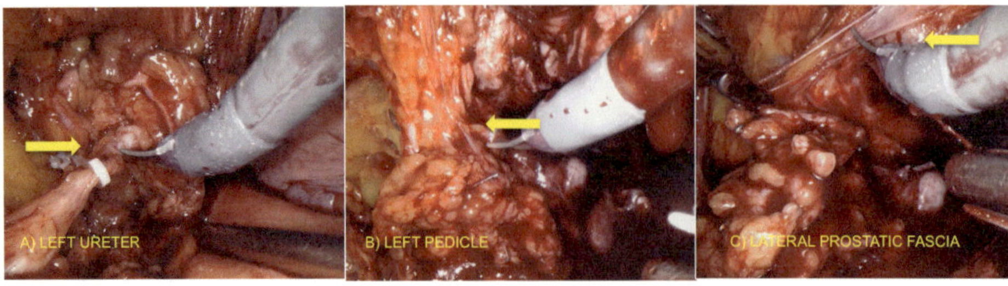

Figure 10.
Left side ureter and prostate fascia.

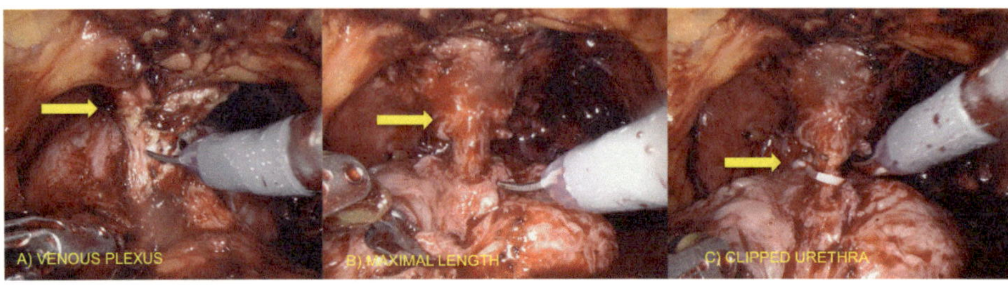

Figure 11.
Endopelvic fascia and ligaments preserved.

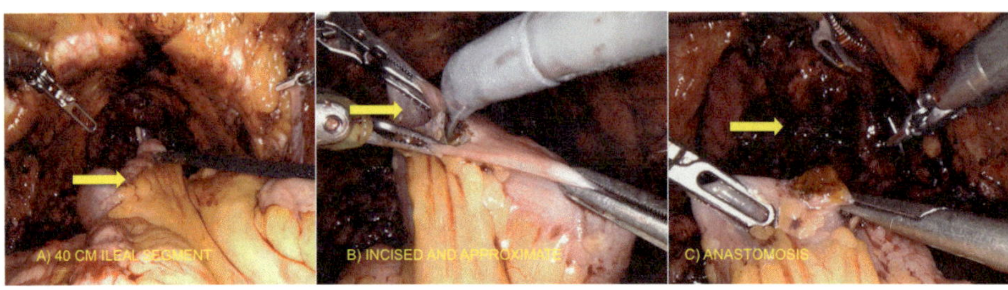

Figure 12.
Ileal segment and urethra-ileal anastomosis.

creation goes by selecting a 40 cm ileal segment form 15 to 20 cm proximal to the ileocecal valve. The segment is arranged in a modified Y shape [22]. The ileal segment is approximate to the urethra for an anastomosis (**Figure 12**).

The continuity of the bowel is achieved with a latero-lateral ileal anastomosis. Our group prefers to use a robotic Da Vinci system stapler, if not available, a laparoscopic stapler could be used trough the 15 mm assistant-trocar (**Figure 13**).

Detubularization of the bowel starts for the two ileal limbs in the antimesenteric border. Construction of the posterior plate is performed by suturing the medial edges of the detubularized limbs (**Figure 14**).

The proximal part of the posterior plate is folded anteriorly and suture for the creation of the anterior wall, the lateral windows are closed with running sutures (**Figure 15**) [22, 23].

The ureter is spatulated and implanted over the proximal end of both ileal limbs without antireflux technique independently with two plates running suture (**Figure 16**).

The neobladder is tested by the instillation of 500 cc of saline by the definitive catheter. A drain is place in the left side of the cavity and the specimen is extracted at the end of the procedure via a 5 cm midline incision [22, 23].

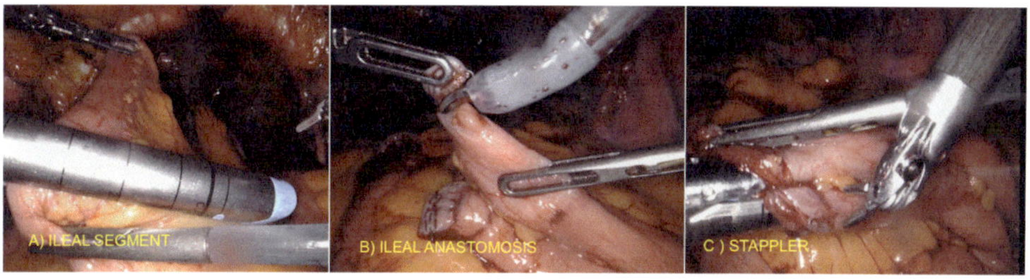

Figure 13.
Latero-lateral ileal anastomosis.

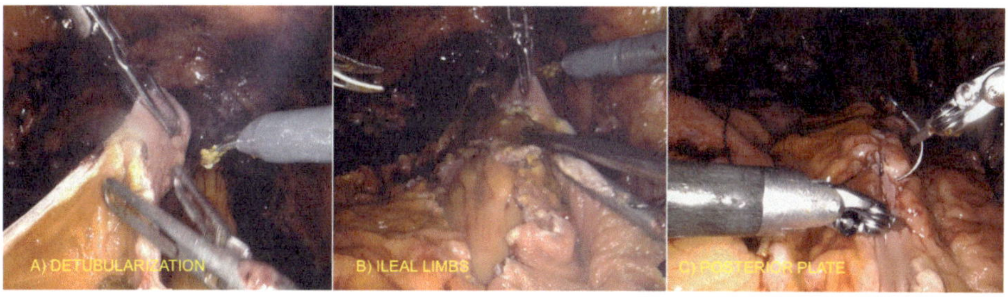

Figure 14.
Detubularization and posterior plate.

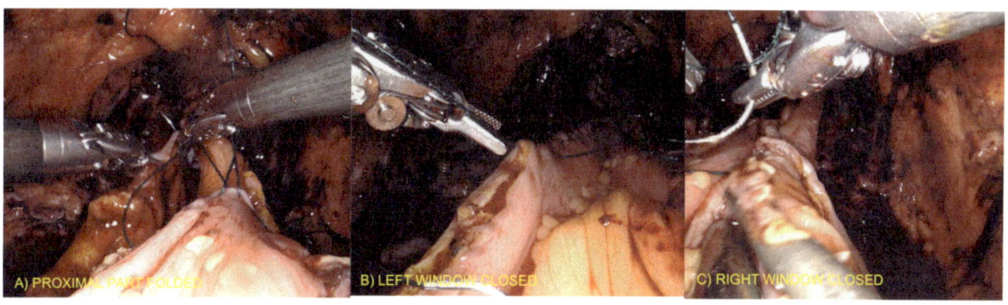

Figure 15.
Proximal part folded. Lateral close to create the neobladder.

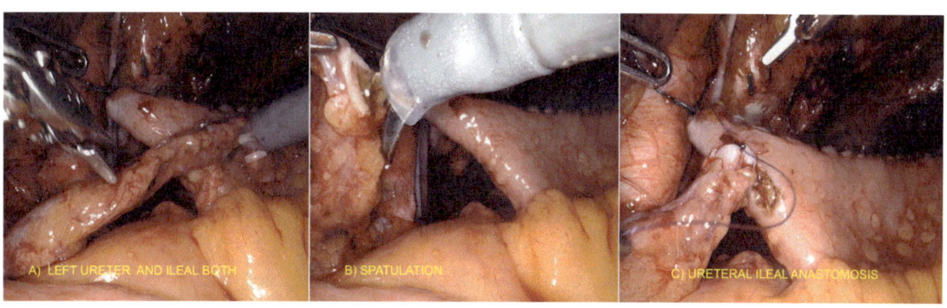

Figure 16.
Ureteral ileal anastomosis.

6. Others techniques for neo-bladder

Some other worldwide groups have developed shaping techniques, equally safe and effective, some of them are resume in the next lines.

The *Karolinska modified Studer "U"*a 55–60 cm ileum is isolated 25 cm proximal to the ileocecal valve. After antimesenteric incision and detubularization the posterior plate is created and its follow by an anterior closure using the initial 15 cm approximately. The rest of the segment is part of the chimney and in his lower side proximal to the pouch is kept open to stend the ureters later. The uretero-ileal anastomosis is perform in the free-top of the chimney once the Simple J ureteric stents were previously introduce [22, 23].

The *Padua Intracorporeal Neo-Bladder* starts with a segment of 42 cm portion of the ileum, detubularization of the distal part 8 cm is perform, follow by detubularization of the distal side 24 cm, the left horn is created with a stapler. The first 8 cm ileum segment is folded and sutured to the first 8 cm ileum segment, creating the posterior plate. To complete the anterior wall, the last 16 cm of the posterior plate are folded to configure it, both edges are suture together. The urethro-ileal anastomosis is performed and the uretero-ieal anastomosis is performed over the posterior wall [23].

The *modified Studer "U"* from University of Southern California, starts with the identification of the most mobile terminal ileum to reach the urethra. 11 cm towards the ileocecal valve for distal end of the pouch, 22 cm for apex of the posterior plate. 44 cm for proximal end of the pouch and beginning of the chimney. The distribution goes to bowel detubularization, creation of the posterior plate and rotation 90o counterclockwise. Urethto – ileal anastomosis and cross folding of the pouch is perform. The uretero ileal anastomosis is performed end-to-side [24].

The *Hautmann W*, a 50 cm of the ileum is isolated and divided into a right and left limb, then the ileum is detubularized and suture to create the posterior plate by and ascending and descending loop. Urethro-ileal anastomosis is performed by a tension-free Van Velthoven technique. The half of the anterior wall is closure and uretero ileal anastomosis is made on each chimney once the ureters were spatulated [22, 23].

The *Pyramid Pouch* starts with the selection of a 50 cm segment of the ileum > 15 cm proximal to the ileocecal valve. The utethral-ileal anastomosis is done at this point, following by the detubularization and formation of the posterior plate except the 2 cm uppermost portion as chimneys. 10 cm of the anterior plate are closure to accomplish the anterior wall. Uretero-ileal anastomosis an end-to-side is performed over the proximal end of both ileal limbs [22, 23].

7. Literature review

The benefits of robotic-assisted laparoscopic surgery rely mainly on the enhancement implied to the ergonomics of the surgeon and a reduction of the learning curve for some procedures. The down size is the lack of tactile feedback during the procedure and the associated costs. Specific improvements to robotic-assisted radical cystectomy are decreased intra-operative blood loss, reduced blood transfusion rates and a shorter length of hospital stay days. Due to the minimally invasive procedure, the surgical time have a tendency to increase in the robotic approach radical cystectomy.

Menon et al. was the first to describe a nerve-sparing robotic-assisted radical cysto-prostatectomy and extra-corporeal urinary diversion back in 2003 [10]. The completely intra-corporeal urinary diversion was reported by Gill et al. in the year 2000. The intra-corporeal urinary diversion was performed in a laparoscopic radical cystectomy and since then the technique found it's way to more recent robotic procedures [25]. The robotic-assisted radical cystectomy (RARC) continues to evolve and the first randomized controlled trial comparing it with open radical cystectomy (ORC) was published in 2009 [26]. The international literature includes multiple articles of technique and complications of RARC but a scarce number of randomized controlled trials comparing its oncologic outcomes and/or benefits with a different approach.

As previously mentioned, the first randomized controlled trial (RCT) to confirm the viability and oncologic safety of the RARC in comparison to ORC was published by Nix in 2009. Nix and his group found a median surgical time longer for RARC, lesser intra-operative blood loss, shorter time to bowel sounds and shorter hospital stay in comparison with ORC [26]. In contrast, controversial findings have been reported comparing RARC and ORC. A meta-analysis of the RCT's found no significant difference in peri-operative complications, length of hospital stay, time to flatus, lymph node yield and positive surgical margins [27]. A lower intra-operative blood loss and longer surgical time is a consistency among the studies.

Comparative findings (surgical, peri-operative complications and oncologic) between randomized controlled trials are described (**Table 1**).

7.1 Oncologic results and safety of the robotic-assisted approach

The Robot-assisted radical cystectomy versus open radical cystectomy trial (RAZOR) is a phase 3 non-inferiority study to compare the oncologic outcomes, complications, pelvic nodes burden, cost and morbidity [29]. At the beginning 350 patients were randomized but only 150 patients underwent RARC and 152 patients ORC after exclusions. The 2-year progression-free survival was 72.3% (95% CI 64.3–78.8) in the RARC group and 71.6% (95% CI 63.3–78.2) in the ORC group, these results demonstrated non-inferiority of robotic surgery VS open approach (difference 0.7%, 95% CI −9.6–10.9%, p non-inferiority=0.001). Local recurrences were similar in both groups (RARC 4%, ORC 3%). Twenty two percent and 23% had distant metastasis in RARC and ORC respectively and no port-site recurrences were reported [29]. Results from the International Robotic Cystectomy Consortium confirmed 16% in distant disease-recurrence, 11% local disease-recurrence, 1% peritoneal carcinomatosis and 0.4% port site recurrence [30].

In a RCT update from the Memorial Sloan Kettering Cancer Center, no statistical differences were reported in disease-recurrence (p=0.4), cancer-specific survival (p=0.4) and overall-survival (p=0.8) between RARC and ORC groups. The authors reported a median follow-up of 4.9 years [31].

In a recent meta-analysis, the disease-recurrence was analyzed in 458 patients with no difference between RARC and ORC (RR 0.94, 95% CI 0.69–1.29) [32]. In the same study, all included articles reported the rate of positive surgical margins (PSM) of 541 participants, it stated no difference between a robotic and open approach (RR 1.16, 95% CI 0.56–2.40) [32]. Tang et al. pooled data from 3 different RCTs and his collaborative group reported that both approaches have similar rate of PSM [33]. A Cochrane review found similar outcomes in the time-to-recurrence and PSM rates for both surgical approaches [34].

The CORAL trial update described similar five-year survival for open, robotic-assisted and laparoscopic radical cystectomy. The 5-year recurrence-free survival was 60%, 58% and 71%; 5-year cancer-specific survival was 64%, 68% and 69%; and 5-year overall survival was 55%, 61% and 61% for open, robotic-assisted and laparoscopic radical cystectomy, respectively [35].

7.2 Operative time

The RARC operative time has been reported to be the longer in comparison to the open approach, with a mean difference from 68.51–90 minutes [32, 36, 37]. Tang et al.

	Nix et al. [26] n (%) OR mean (range)		Bochner et al. [28] n (%) OR median (range)		Parekh et al. [29] n (%) OR median (range)	
	⁺RARC (21)	**ꞔORC (20)**	**⁺RARC (60)**	**ꞔORC (58)**	**⁺RARC (150)**	**ꞔORC (152)**
Age, *years-old*	67.4 (33–81)	69.2 (51–80)	66 (60–71)	65 (58–69)	70 (43–90)	67 (37–85)
Men/Women	14 (67)/7 (33)	17 (85)/3 (15)	51 (85)/15 (15)	42 (72)/16 (28)	126 (84%)/24 (16%)	128 (84%)/24 (16%)
Body Mass Index, kg/m^2	27.5	28.4	27.9	29	27.8	28.2
Neoadjuvant Chemotherapy	*	*	19 (32)	26 (45)	41 (27%)	55 (36%)
Surgical blood loss, *mL*	258	575	516 (*mean*)	676 (*mean*)	300 (200–500)	700 (500–1000)
Surgical Complications						
None	14 (67)	10 (50)	23 (38)	20 (34)	49 (33)	47 (31)
Clavien Dindo I-II	5 (28)	7 (35)	24 (40)	26 (45)	68 (45)	71 (47)
Clavien-Dindo III-V	2 (5)	3 (15)	13 (22)	12 (21)	33 (22)	34 (22)
Urinary diversion	extracorporeal	—	extracorporeal	—	extracorporeal	—
T Stage	*TxN+: 4 (19)*	*TxN+: 7 (35)*				
T0			13 (22)	7 (12)	22 (15)	31 (20)
Ta, Tis			15 (24.7)	14 (24.2)	25 (17)	25 (16)
T1	T0-T2: 14 (67)	T0-T2: 8 (40)	7 (12)	11 (19)	19 (13)	15 (10)
T2			8 (13)	7 (12)	38 (25)	33 (22)
T3	T3-T4: 3 (14)	T3-T4: 5 (25)	12 (20)	15 (26)	35 (23)	32 (21)
T4a/T4b			5 (8.3)	4 (6.9)	10 (6)/1 (1)	14 (9)/3 (2)
Length of stay, *days*	5.1	6	8 (*mean*)	8 (*mean*)	6 (5–10)	7 (6–10)
Surgical time, *min*	252	212	456 (*mean*)	329 (*mean*)	428 (322–509)	361 (281–450)
Extended lymph node dissection	21	20	13 (22)	26 (45)	76/149 (51%)	84/152 (55%)

DOI: http://dx.doi.org/10.5772/intechopen.98973

	Nix et al. [26] *n* **(%) OR mean (range)**		**Bochner et al. [28]** *n* **(%) OR median (range)**		**Parekh et al. [29]** *n* **(%) OR median (range)**	
	+RARC (21)	**ςORC (20)**	**+RARC (60)**	**ςORC (58)**	**+RARC (150)**	**ςORC (152)**
Lymph nodes resected	19 (12–30)	18 (8–30)	31.9 (*mean*)	30 (*mean*)	23.3 (12.5%)	25.7 (14.5%)
Positive surgical margins	0	0	2 (3.6)	3 (4.8)	9 (6%)	7 (5%)

+*Robotic-assisted radical cystectomy.*
ς*Open radical cystectomy.*
**Not mentioned.*

Table 1.
Comparative findings between randomized controlled trials.

meta-analysis also reported a longer surgical time in comparison to ORC [33]. A prolonged operative time could be associated to peri-operative complications, such as, deep vein thrombosis, wound infection and increase anesthetic risk [32].

7.3 Urinary diversion

In a retrospectively study of 2,125 patients, Hussein et al. reported the outcomes of 1,094 patients who underwent RARC with intra-corporeal urinary diversion (ICUD) [38]. ICUD was associated with a shorter surgical time (357 VS 400 minutes, $p<0.001$), less surgical blood loss (300 VS 350 mL, $p<0.001$) and fewer blood transfusions (5% VS 13%, $p<0.001$) than extra-corporeal urinary diversion (ECUD) but high-grade complications were more frequent (57% VS 43%) 30 days after surgery. The incidence of high-grade complications decreased significantly trough time, from 25% in 2005 to 6% in 2015 (p<0.001) and remained stable [38]. The ICUD is very complex robotic procedure but the decision to perform a type of urinary diversion (neo-bladder o cutaneous pouch) should not be based on the surgical approach [18].

The modified Y-neo-bladder intra-corporeal technique performed in the Clinique Saint-Augustin, described by Asimakopoulos and two of the authors of this chapter, is an almost spherical urinary reservoir without the need to transpose either ureter [19]. This will allow the neobladder to remain aligned in a natural fashion and enables a tension-free ureter-neo-bladder anastomosis (buttonhole anastomosis). The reported data obtained via voiding charts indicated low 12-month voiding frequency with no pathological post-void residual volume, good mean maximal functional bladder capacity and no need for clean intermittent catheterization [19].

7.4 Complications

Previously, multiple articles and reviews have stated a lower rate of peri-operative complications related RARC [37]. The RCT elaborated by Bochner et al. described a rate of peri-operative complications grade 2–5 (Clavien-Dindo) of 62% for RARC and 66% for ORC [39]. In accordance with those findings, a recent RCT meta-analysis found similar peri-operative complication rate for RARC and ORC within 30 days [33]. Sathianathen et al. and Khan et al. meta-analysis, reported no difference in the 90-day incidence of major complications (Clavien Dindo III-V) between both approaches (RR 1.06, CI 95% 0.75–1.49) [32, 37].

One key benefit of the robotic surgery is lower surgical blood loss (mean difference of 300 mL), it is possible to suggest that RARC may reduce the rate of transfusion [32–34, 36]. In contrast, multiple articles have reported no difference in the rate of blood transfusion and others up to 77% reduction in the odds for blood transfusion [24, 26]. Wang et al. reported an estimated median blood loss of 400 (100–1200) mL for RARC and 750 (250–2500) mL for ORC (p=0–002), 0.5 (0–3) and 2 (0–7) units of blood for transfusion respectively (p=0.007) [36].

Sathianathen meta-analysis included two studies that reported the blood transfusion rate as a result, the peri-operative blood transfusion necessity was lower for RARC (42% risk reduction) [32]. As previously mentioned, an odds reduction of blood transfusion might be one of the benefits of the robotic approach because of the clinical impact, risks and adverse effects of blood transfusions should not be foreseen (hemolysis, anaphylaxis).

7.5 Length of hospital stay

n the article of Wang and his group, the median length of hospital stay days for RARC was 5 (4–18) days and 8 (5–28) days for ORC (p=0.007) [36]. The length of stay <5 days for the RARC group was 40/139 (29%) and 27/146 (18%) for ORC group (p=0.0407) [29]. The length of stay had no statistical difference in the analysis of Tang and his group (weighted mean difference: −0.60, 95% CI: −1.61–0.40, p=.24) [33]. Sathianathen et al. also reported a minimal marginal and no statistical difference in length of stay for the RARC group (RR −0.63, CI 95% −1.21−−0.05) [32].

7.6 Learning curve/surgeon volume

The International Robotic Cystectomy Consortium reported a learning curve of twenty-one robotic procedures to achieve a surgical time cutoff of 390 minutes. In contrast, a learning curve of more than 30 procedures was required for a PSM rate below 5%. Beyond 50 cases an improvement in the surgeon's performance (a decrease mean operative time and a higher lymph node yield) has been seen [28, 32, 40].

8. Conclusion

The robot-assisted cystectomy for the male or female with the intra-corporeal urinary diversion is a feasible technique and safe in experienced surgeon hands. There exist different types of intra-corporeal neo-bladders. The "Y" neo-bladder technical aspects of this procedure are part of the arsenal to choose. The results between open radical cystectomy and robotic need more studies to improve the data and the real results for the upgrade of the procedure. There is not yet enough evidence in the literature, even if the actual results are promising.

Conflict of interest

The authors declare no conflict of interest.

Notes/Thanks/Other Declarations

Thanks to collaborative group, and special thanks to who provided linguistic revision.

Nomenclature

RARC	robot-assisted radical cystectomy
ORC	open radical cystectomy
RC	radical cystectomy
NB	neo bladder
RCT	randomized controlled trial
ICUD	intra-corporeal urinary diversion
ECUD	extra-corporeal urinary diversion
IRCC	international robotic cystectomy consortium

Author details

Víctor Enrique Corona-Montes[1,2]*, Eduardo Gonzalez-Cuenca[2], Laurent López[3], Juan Eduardo Sánchez-Núñez[2] and Richard Gaston[3]

1 American British Cowdray Medical Center (A.B.C.), México City, México

2 Uro-Oncology Department, General Hospital of Mexico, México City, México

3 Department of Urology, Clinique Saint Augustin, Bordeaux, France

*Address all correspondence to: urocorona@hotmail.com

References

[1] Lenis AT, Lec PM, Chamie K, Mshs M. Bladder Cancer: A Review. JAMA. 2020;324(19):1980-1991. DOI:10.1001/jama.2020.17598

[2] Liss MA, Kader AK. Robotic-assisted laparoscopic radical cystectomy: history, techniques and outcomes. World J Urol. 2013;31(3):489-97. DOI:10.1007/s00345-013-1053-z

[3] Ghoneim MA, Abdel-Latif M, el-Mekresh M, Abol-Enein H, Mosbah A, Ashamallah A, et al. Radical cystectomy for carcinoma of the bladder: 2,720 consecutive cases 5 years later. J Urol. 2008;180(1):121-7. DOI:10.1016/j.uro.2008.03.024

[4] Yates DR, Vaessen C, Roupret M. From Leonardo to da Vinci: the history of robot-assisted surgery in urology. BJU Int. 2011;108(11):1708-13; discussion 1714. DOI:10.1111/j.1464-410X.2011.10576.x

[5] Marshall VJ, Whitemore WF. A technique for the extension of radical surgery in the treatment of vesical cancer. Cancer. 1949;2(3):424-8. DOI:10.1002/1097-0142(194905)2:3<424::aid-cncr2820020306>3.0.co;2-y

[6] Otero JR, Paparel P, Atreya D, Touijer K, Guillonneau B. History, evolution and application of robotic surgery in urology. Arch Esp Urol. 2007;60(4):335-41. DOI:10.4321/s0004-06142007000400002.

[7] Murphy DG, Challacombe BJ, Elhage O, O'Brien TS, Rimington P, Khan MS, et al. Robotic-assisted Laparoscopic Radical Cystectomy with Extracorporeal Urinary Diversion: Initial Experience. Eur Urol. 2008;54(3):570-80. DOI:10.1016/j.eururo.2008.04.011.

[8] Knox ML, El-Galley R, Busby JE. Robotic versus Open Radical Cystectomy: identification of patients who benefit from the robotic approach. J Endourol. 2013;27(1):40-4. DOI:10.1089/end.2012.0168.

[9] Ng CK, Kauffman EC, Lee M-M, Otto BJ, Portnoff A, Ehrlich JR, et al. A Comparison of postoperative complications in Open versus Robotic Cystectomy. Eur Urol. 2010;57(2):274-81. DOI: 10.1016/j.eururo.2009.06.001.

[10] Menon M, Hemal AK, Tewari A, Shrivastava A, Shoma AM, El-Tabey NA, et al. Nerve-sparing robot-assisted radical cystoprostatectomy and urinary diversion. BJU International 2003;92:232-6. DOI:10.1046/j.1464-410x.2003.04329.x.

[11] Bhandari M, Menon M. Prostatectomía radical robótica: técnica del Vattikuti Institute Prostatectomy (VIP) y resultados actuales. Arch Esp Urol 2007;60(4):397-407. DOI:10.4321/S0004-06142007000400010

[12] Parra RO, Andrus CH, Jones JP, Boullier JA. Laparoscopic Cystectomy: Initial Report on a New Treatment for the Retained Bladder. J Urol 1992;148(4):1140-4. DOI:10.1016/s0022-5347(17)36843-x

[13] Sánchez de Badajoz E, Gallego Perales JL, Reche Rosado A, Gutierrez de la Cruz JM, Jimenez Garrido A. Laparoscopic cystectomy and ileal conduit: Case Report. J Endourol. 1995;9(1):59-62. DOI:10.1089/end.1995.9.59

[14] Khan MS. The evolution of robotic cystectomy. BJU Int. 2014;113(2):178. DOI:10.1111/bju.12607

[15] Beecken W-D, Wolfram M, Engl T, Bentas W, Probst M, Blaheta R, Oertl A, et al. Robotic-Assisted laparoscopic radical cystectomy and intra-abdominal

formation of an orthotopic ileal neobladder. Eur Urol. 2003;44(3):337-9. DOI:10.1016/s0302-2838(03)00301-4

[16] Brooks JD, Chao WM, Kerr J. Male pelvic anatomy reconstructed from the visible human data set. J Urol 1998;159(3):868-872. PMID:9474171

[17] Ong K., Herdiman O, Johnson L, Lawrentschuk N. Orthotopic bladder substitution (neobladder): part I: indications, patient selection, preoperative education, and counseling. J Wound Ostomy Continence Nurs. 2013;40(1):73-82. DOI:10.1097/WON.0b013e31827759ea

[18] Witjes JA. Muscle-Invasive and Metastatic Bladder Cancer. European Association of Urology Guidelines [Internet]. 2020. Available from: https://uroweb.org/guideline/bladder-cancer-muscle-invasive-and-metastatic/#1/ [Accessed: 2020-11-02]

[19] Asimakopoulos AD, Campagna A, Gakis G, Corona Montes VE, Piechaud T, Hoepffner J-L, et al. Nerve Sparing, Robot-Assisted Radical Cystectomy with Intracorporeal Bladder Substitution in the Male. J Urol 2016;196(5):1549-57. DOI:10.1016/j.juro.2016.04.114.

[20] Stenzl A, Nagele U, Kuczyk M, Sievert K-D, Anastasiadis A, Seibold J, Corvin S. Cystectomy – Technical Considerations in Male and Female Patients. EAU Update Series 2005;3(3):138-146. DOI: 10.1016/j.euus.2005.07.004

[21] Nagele U, Sievert K-D, Merseburger AS, Anastasiadis AG, Stenzl A. Urinary Diversion Following Cystectomy. EAU Update Series 2005;3(3):129-137. DOI: 10.1016/j.euus.2005.07.003

[22] Otaola-Arca H, Seetharam Bhat KR, Moschovas MC, Orvieto M. Totally intracorporeal robot-assisted urinary diversion for bladder cancer (part 2). Review and detailed characterization of the existing intracorporeal orthotopic ileal neobladder. Asian Journal of Urology. DOI:10.1016/j.ajur.2020.05.013

[23] Otaola-Arca H, Coelho R, Patel VR, Orvieto M. Totally intracorporeal robot-assisted urinary diversion for bladder cancer (Part 1). Review and detailed characterizarion of ilean conduit and modified Indiana pouch. Asian Journal of Urology. DOI:10.1016/j.ajur.2020.10.001

[24] Thress TM, Coolson MS, Patel S. Robotic Cystectomy with Intracorporeal Urinary Diversion: Techniques and Outcomes. Urol Clin North Am. 2018 Feb;45(1):67-77. DOI: 10.1016/j.ucl.2017.09.009.PMIDE: 29169452.

[25] Gill IS, Fergany A, Klein EA, Kaouk JH, Sung GT, Meraney AM, et al. Laparoscopic radical cystoprostatectomy with ileal conduit performed completely intracorporeally: the initial 2 cases. Urology 2000;56:26-9–discussion29-30. DOI:10.1016/s0090-4295(00)00598-7.

[26] Nix J, Smith A, Kurpad R, Nielsen ME, Wallen EM, Pruthi RS. Prospective randomized controlled trial of robotic versus open radical cystectomy for bladder cancer: perioperative and pathologic results. Eur Urol 2010;57:196-201. DOI:10.1016/j.eururo.2009.10.024.

[27] Tang J-Q, Zhao Z, Liang Y, Liao G. Robotic-assisted versus open radical cystectomy in bladder cancer: A meta-analysis of four randomized controlled trails. Int J Med Robot 2018;14. DOI:10.1002/rcs.1867.

[28] Hayn MH, Hussain A, Mansour AM, Andrews PE, Carpentier P, Castle E, et al. The learning curve of robot-assisted radical cystectomy: results from the International Robotic Cystectomy Consortium. Eur Urol 2010;58:197-202. DOI:10.1016/j.eururo.2010.04.024.

[29] Parekh DJ, Reis IM, Castle EP, Gonzalgo ML, Woods ME, Svatek RS, et al. Robot-assisted radical cystectomy versus open radical cystectomy in patients with bladder cancer (RAZOR): an open-label, randomised, phase 3, non-inferiority trial. The Lancet 2018;391:2525-36. DOI:10.1016/S0140-6736(18)30996-6.

[30] Hussein AA, Saar M, May PR, Wijburg CJ, Richstone L, Wagner A, et al. Early Oncologic Failure after Robot-Assisted Radical Cystectomy: Results from the International Robotic Cystectomy Consortium. J Urol 2017;197:1427-36. DOI:10.1016/j.juro.2016.12.048.

[31] Bochner BH, Dalbagni G, Marzouk KH, Sjoberg DD, Lee J, Donat SM, et al. Randomized Trial Comparing Open Radical Cystectomy and Robot-assisted Laparoscopic Radical Cystectomy: Oncologic Outcomes. Eur Urol 2018;74:465-71. DOI:10.1016/j.eururo.2018.04.030.

[32] Sathianathen NJ, Kalapara A, Frydenberg M, Lawrentschuk N, Weight CJ, Parekh D, et al. Robotic Assisted Radical Cystectomy vs Open Radical Cystectomy: Systematic Review and Meta-Analysis. J Urol 2019;201:715-20. DOI:10.1016/j.juro.2018.10.006.

[33] Tang J-Q, Zhao Z, Liang Y, Liao G. Robotic-assisted versus open radical cystectomy in bladder cancer: A meta-analysis of four randomized controlled trails. Int J Med Robot 2018;14. DOI:10.1002/rcs.1867.

[34] Rai BP, Bondad J, Vasdev N, Adshead J, Lane T, Ahmed K, et al. Robotic versus open radical cystectomy for bladder cancer in adults. Cochrane Database Syst Rev 2019;4:CD011903. DOI:10.1002/14651858.CD011903.pub2.

[35] Khan MS, Omar K, Ahmed K, Gan C, Van Hemelrijck M, Nair R, et al. Long-term Oncological Outcomes from an Early Phase Randomised Controlled Three-arm Trial of Open, Robotic, and Laparoscopic Radical Cystectomy (CORAL). Eur Urol 2020;77:110-8. DOI:10.1016/j.eururo.2019.10.027.

[36] Wang GJ, Barocas DA, Raman JD, Scherr DS. Robotic vs open radical cystectomy: prospective comparison of perioperative outcomes and pathological measures of early oncological efficacy. BJU International 2008;101:89-93. DOI:10.1111/j.1464-410X.2007.07212.x.

[37] Khan MS, Gan C, Ahmed K, Ismail AF, Watkins J, Summers JA, et al. A Single-centre Early Phase Randomised Controlled Three-arm Trial of Open, Robotic, and Laparoscopic Radical Cystectomy (CORAL). Eur Urol 2016;69:613-21. DOI:10.1016/j.eururo.2015.07.038.

[38] Hussein AA, May PR, Jing Z, Ahmed YE, Wijburg CJ, Canda AE, et al. Outcomes of Intracorporeal Urinary Diversion after Robot-Assisted Radical Cystectomy: Results from the International Robotic Cystectomy Consortium. J Urol 2018;199:1302-11. DOI:10.1016/j.juro.2017.12.045.

[39] Bochner BH, Dalbagni G, Sjoberg DD, Silberstein J, Paz GEK, Donat SM, et al. Comparing Open Radical Cystectomy and Robot-assisted Laparoscopic Radical Cystectomy: A Randomized Clinical Trial. Eur Urol 2015;67:1042-50. DOI:10.1016/j.eururo.2014.11.043.

[40] May D, Gills J, Delacroix SE. Robotic Cystectomy. Urol Clin North Am 2018;45:183-8. DOI:10.1016/j.ucl.2017.12.012.

Chapter 5

Robotic Orthotopic Neobladder: The Two Chimney Technique

Panagiotis Pardalidis, Nikolaos Andriopoulos and Nikolaos Pardalidis

Abstract

Bladder substitution following radical cystectomy for urothelial cancer (transitional cell carcinoma) has become increasingly common and in many centers has evolved to become the standard method of urinary diversion. Orthotopic neobladder has been a commonly used option for urinary diversion since the 1980s. Advantages of this type of diversion are the ability to avoid an ostomy, voiding function similar to the native bladder, and improved cosmesis. Robotic intracorporeal neobladder creation has demonstrated similar outcomes to open technique and represents a promising minimally invasive diversion for the future. The Studer pouch is widely used nowadays, yet there are still some drawbacks. Therefore, we designed a technique that would offer an orthotopic ureteroileal anastomosis by using a two chimney modification. This modification is simple to handle, safe and free of ureteric stricture or reflux. With low stricture rates, this modified procedure of ureterointestinal anastomosis, is worthy of further promotion.

Keywords: urothelial bladder cancer, urinary diversion, bladder substitution, robotic orthotopic neobladder, ureteroileal anastomosis

1. Introduction

Indications for orthotopic diversion are: absence of malignancy of the prostatic urethra in men or the bladder neck in women, adequate renal function (GFR >35–40), normal liver function, absence of severe urethral stricture disease, absence of inflammatory bowel disease (IBD) and a reliable patient with good mental status and dexterity. Drawbacks unique to a neobladder include urinary incontinence, incomplete emptying, need for self-intermittent catheterization (SIC) and longer operative times. Many viable surgical techniques exist and offer good functional and oncological outcomes. In determining the best type of urinary diversion for a specific patient, consideration must be given to both the morbidity associated with surgery and the potential positive impact on the patient's quality of life.

Kock demonstrated the importance of complete detubularization of the bowel segment and the double-folding technique that creates the most spheric shape possible (Kock, 1982). These concepts are the cornerstone of current cutaneous and orthotopic reservoirs [1].

In 1979, Camey and Le Duc reported their pioneering clinical experience with orthotopic substitution to the native urethra in male bladder cancer patients (Camey and Le Duc, 1979). The initial Camey diversion used an intact segment of ileum, resulting in a high-pressure reservoir. Subsequently the Camey II detubularized reservoir (Camey, 1990); Hautmann W-neobladder (Hautmann, 1988); "hemi-Kock" neobladder (Skinner, 1991); Studer pouch (Studer, 1989); extraserosal-lined ureteral tunnel (Abol-Enein and Ghoneim, 1993); T pouch (Stein, 1998); stomach neobladder (Hauri, 1998); cecal and ileocecal neobladders (Light and Engelmann, 1986; Mansson and Colleen, 1990); and sigmoid reservoir (Reddy and Lange, 1987) have all been described [1]. All those techniques of urinary diversion have been evaluated through time, providing good renal preservation as well as functional and oncologic outcomes. Orthotopic diversion quickly surpassed continent cutaneous diversion in popularity for both patients and physicians because it allows natural voiding, is simpler to construct and is less likely to require revision surgery at a later date.

Although the ideal bladder substitute remains to be developed, the orthotopic neobladder most closely resembles the original bladder in both location and function. This form of lower urinary tract reconstruction relies on the intact external rhabdosphincter continence mechanism, seldom requires intermittent catheterization and avoids the difficulties associated with the efferent continence mechanism of continent cutaneous reservoirs. Voiding is accomplished by relaxation of the pelvic floor musculature (as in normal voiding) along with a concomitant increase in intra-abdominal pressure (Valsalva maneuver).

It is estimated that approximately 80–90% of male patients and 75% of female patients undergoing cystectomy are potential candidates for neobladder construction from a purely medical standpoint.

2. Historic evolution of orthotopic urinary diversion

Three types of urinary diversion have been developed until now: conduit diversion, continent cutaneous diversion and the latest orthotopic diversion (**Figure 1**).

Both ileal and colon conduits present with long term complications such as peristomal hernia, pyelonephritis, stomal stenosis and renal deterioration. Likewise, continent cutaneous diversions relate with malfunction of the efferent continence mechanism and therefore, open surgical revision is often required.

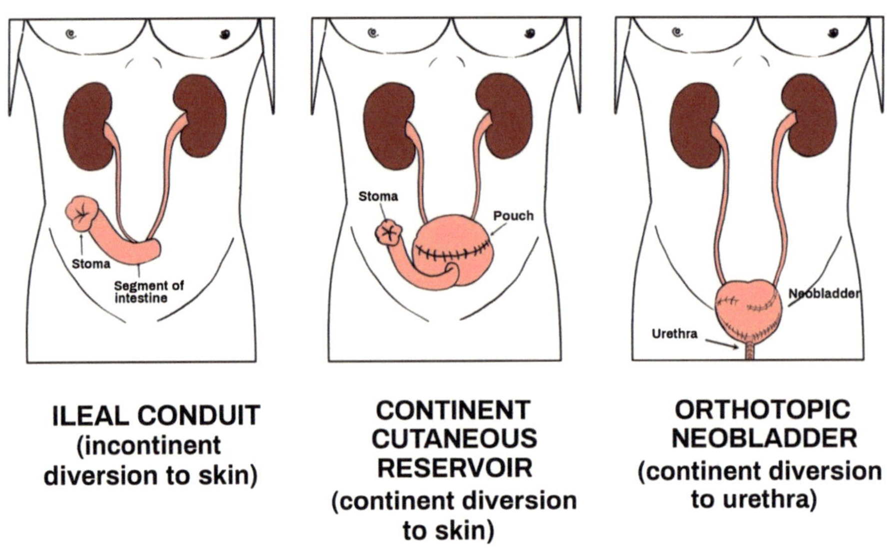

Figure 1.
Types of urinary diversion.

On the contrary, patients with orthotopic neobladder formation are able to void to completion without the need of intermittent catheterization, because the mechanism of continence relies on the rhabdosphincter.

3. Basic principles of continent orthotopic urinary diversion

In order to construct a functional orthotopic neobladder using intestinal segment, three basic principles must be satisfied.

First of all, the urethra of the patient must not be obstructed and must have adequate external sphincter mechanism.

Second, the reservoir must be sufficiently compliant to maintain a low pressure during the filling phase. This is best achieved by opening the bowel segment longitudinally to completely detubularize it and folding it to create a spheric shape.

The shape of the neobladder is of great importance. The sphere seems to be the best choice as it has the greatest internal volume and therefore the greatest capacity.

In addition, the Kock pouch and also S and W shaped reservoirs maintain low internal pressures throughout the filling phase, due to low pressure contractions of the bowel wall.

All current continent diversion techniques use detubularized bowel to construct the reservoir.

Third, the reservoir must have adequate volume to allow for reasonable voiding intervals. In general, this should be at least 300 to 500 mL once the pouch is mature.

The standard 44-cm length of ileum formed into a double-folding reservoir by the Kock technique (also used for both the Studer and T pouch neobladders) has an initial capacity of less than 200 mL but within the first year stretches to hold 500 to 600 mL at low pressure [1].

In general, small bowel, when available, has advantages over colon in terms of wall compliance and ability to stretch, as well as reduced mucous formation.

4. Techniques for orthotopic bladder substitution

Reservoirs made of detubularized ileum or ileum and colon together, appear to have the greatest compliance and lowest likelihood of generating intermittent high-pressure contractions.

The circular muscle layer of ileum was found to be most distensible, and the urodynamic characteristics of the ileum appear to be superior to those of the colon.

According to Schrier, ileum neobladders have the larger capacity, lower pressures and better compliance. Likewise, small bowel mesentery has the greatest mobility and can reach to the urethra without much tension [1].

Furthermore, another advantage of the ileum is the intestinal mucosa atrophy, due to the chronic exposure to urine. As a result, mucous production is decreased as well as reabsorption of urinary electrolytes. Mucosal atrophy appears to be more frequent in small bowel reservoirs.

Isolation of the segment of bowel to be used for the diversion must be performed carefully to preserve blood supply to the pouch, as well as to the bowel anastomosis.

The addition of an antireflux mechanism does not appear to be necessary for preservation of the upper tracts and prevention of infections, at least in the intermediate term [2].

5. Surgical techniques

5.1 Ileal reservoirs

For the creation of most ileal reservoirs a 60–75 cm of terminal ileum is used. The segment is detubularized and folded in various ways to create a sphere shape. Several modifications exist regarding the folding technique and variations in the placement of the ureters (with or without antireflux mechanism).

Of the two most popular configurations around the world are the Hautmann W-neobladder (and its various modifications) and the Studer pouch neobladder. Both are relatively simple constructions and allow direct ureteroileal anastomosis, which has been shown to have the lowest risk of subsequent stricture.

5.2 Studer pouch

Studer and colleagues initially described an ileal bladder substitute, as a long, afferent, isoperistaltic, tubular ileal segment. It is believed that the long segment functionally prevents vesicoureteral reflux when the patient voids by Valsalva maneuver (Studer, 1996) [1]. It is straightforward to construct and has become one of the most popular form of orthotopic diversion in the Urological community. The advantages of this bladder substitute include the simplicity of construction, the lack of a requirement for surgical staples and the ability to accommodate short ureters. The reservoir portion uses the optimal double-folded U configuration as originally described by Kock (Kock, 1989). Studer's group reported on 480 of these procedures performed from 1985 through 2005 with excellent long-term results in terms of continence, preservation of renal function and a ureteroileal stricture rate of less than 3% (Studer, 2006). The original description used a 20-cm afferent segment with 40 cm used for the reservoir. In more recent years Studer has advocated using a somewhat shorter afferent ileal segment with similar results (Studer, 2006) [1].

For Studer reservoir creation, a 54 cm of the terminal ileum is isolated, approximately 15-20 cm from the ileocecal valve. The distal and proximal segments are divided in an avascular plane, with staplers, ensuring mobility of the pouch and small bowel anastomosis to the urethra. In the process the Studer pouch is formed in a U shape using 40-44 cm of distal ileum with each limb measuring 20 cm and a proximal 15 cm segment is used as the afferent limb. The proximal end is closed with absorbable sutures, whereas the distal ileal segment is opened 2 cm away from the mesentery and the incised ileal mucosa is oversewn in two layers, using a running 3–0 polyglycolic acid suture for the creation of the sphere.

The rate of ureteroileal stricture is influenced by the type of anastomosis. The direct end-to-side Leadbetter or the combined Wallace anastomoses with interrupted fine absorbable sutures have been shown to have the lowest risk of stricture, approximately 3–6% (Pantuck, 2000; Hautmann, 2011) [1].

Common observations from series of patients undergoing orthotopic diversion include a gradual period of improvement in daytime continence over the first 6 to 12 months with a slower improvement in night-time continence even into the second year.

The evaluation and management of urinary incontinence after orthotopic diversion should be delayed until the neobladder has had time to expand. This may take 6 months to a year after surgery.

6. The robotic cystectomy and two chimney approach

The robot-assisted surgical approach for pelvic urologic oncology has existed since the mid-2000s and the technique for robot-assisted radical cystectomy (RARC) with lymph node dissection has been established. Early oncologic outcomes after RARC and lymph node dissection are safe and efficacious (Hellenthal, 2011) [1]. Moreover, we observed decreased robotic surgery-related complications and improved outcomes over time in our early series (Pardalidis 2011) [3]. Several perceived advantages of robot-assisted approaches for bladder cancer include less pain, minimal blood loss and earlier return of bowel function, which ultimately help in a quicker return to previous quality of life (Challacombe et al., 2011) [1]. Despite smaller incisions and advances in extirpation, recovery has relied mainly on return of bowel function. More than 1700 cases of RARC have been registered in the International Robotic Cystectomy Consortium database (IRCC). Based on data published in 2013 from the IRCC, approximately 18% of procedures have been performed with the complete intracorporeal approach (Ahmed, 2014) [1]. Two commonly performed procedures with the complete intracorporeal approach include the ileal conduit and a modified Studer neobladder.

When constructing orthotopic bladder substitution, a design with features similar to that of a normal bladder must be adopted, including creating a low pressure pouch with adequate capacity and effective preservation of renal function. Controversy still remains regarding the optimal mode of ureteroileal anastomosis. Anti-reflux techniques can be harmful to renal function due to the development of anastomotic strictures at a higher rate than with refluxing techniques (9–20% vs. 1–6%). Refluxing techniques, are easier to perform with a lower stenosis rate in the long-term follow-up period; but these techniques also have drawbacks for renal function, including recurrent pyelonephritis and hydronephrosis caused by vesico-ureteral reflux, especially during voiding due to increasing bladder luminal pressure.

ICUD-EAU International Consultation on Bladder Cancer 2012 does not recommend applying antireflux anastomosis in orthotopic bladder substitutions. Studer

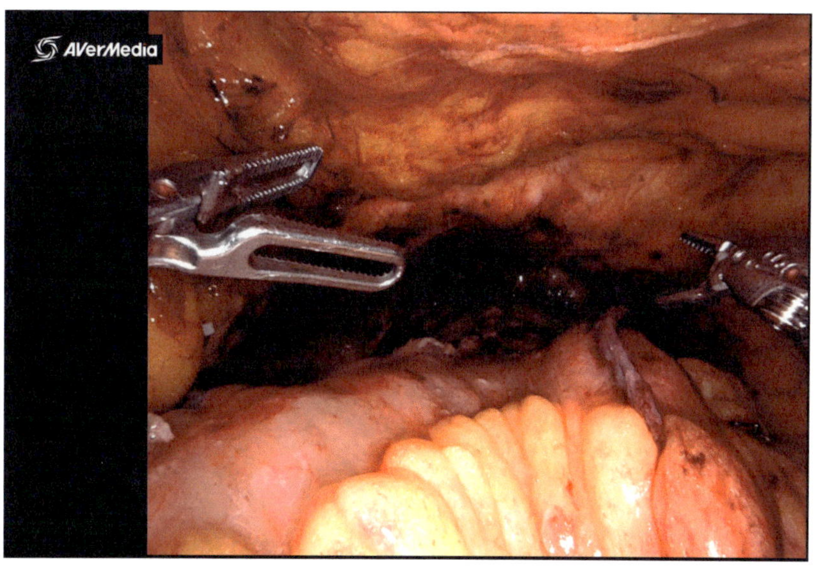

Figure 2.
Two chimney neobladder formation before ureteroneobladder anastomosis.

and Timmer recommend antireflux techniques only in cases where urine diversion can generate great intraluminal pressure and/or when there is a risk of permanent bacterial colonization [2]. Hence, we designed a technique that would resolve these problems by using a two chimney method of ureteroileal anastomosis in an ileal-modified orthotopic bladder substitution.

The Studer pouch is widely used these days, yet there are still some drawbacks. The afferent limb of the Studer pouch is anastomosed with the bilateral ureters together, either in a Wallace I or II fashion so as the left ureter should be tunneled under the mesosigmoid for anastomosis with the afferent ileal segment. This maneuver may be the cause of increased left stenosis occurred twice as frequently as on the right side because of extensive dissection and possible tension creating ischemia of the distal ureteral end. Our technique by formation of two chimneys on each neobladder lateral side and end to end ureteroileal anastomosis, effectively avoids these drawbacks because of the separate bilateral ureteroileal anastomosis. Each ureter is spatulated and anastomosed without tension and less ischemia, so the risk of stenosis is decreased (**Figures 2–11**).

This surgical modification seems to preserve ureteral vascularization, resulting to low stricture rate (4%). Additionally, in case of reintervention it is easier

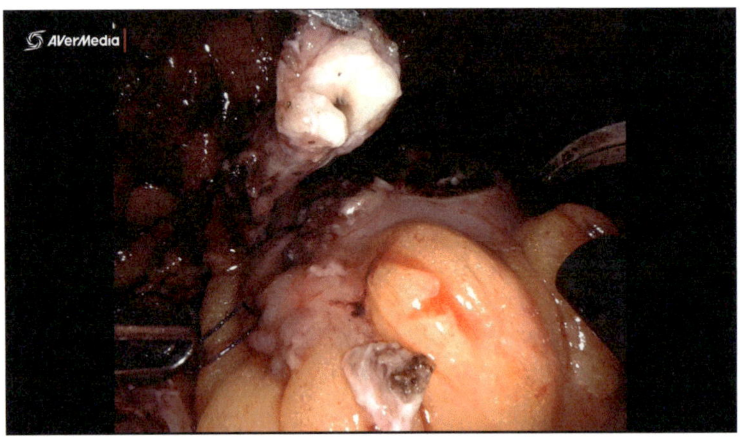

Figure 3.
Spatulation of the left ureter before ureteroneobladder anastomosis.

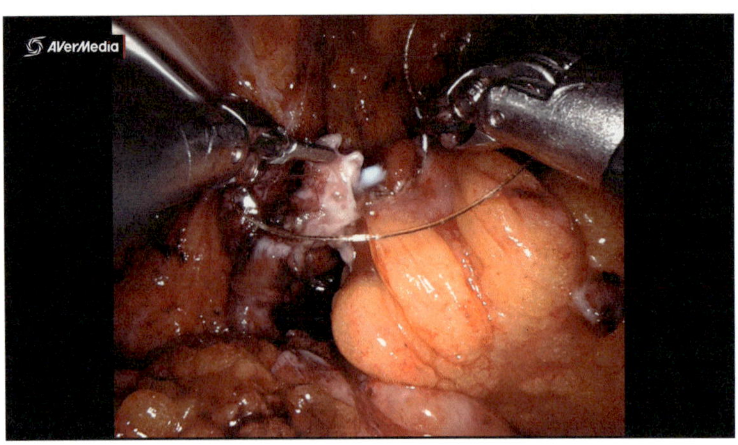

Figure 4.
Left end-to-end ureteroneobladder anastomosis.

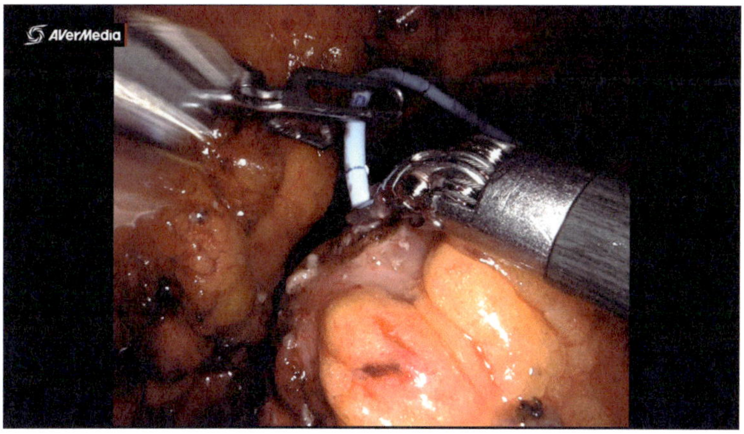

Figure 5.
Ureteral stent catheterization of the left ureter.

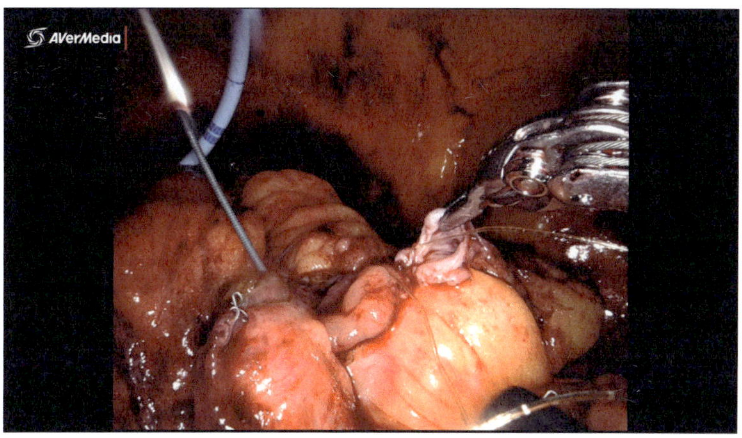

Figure 6.
Right chimney end-to-end ureteroneobladder anastomosis.

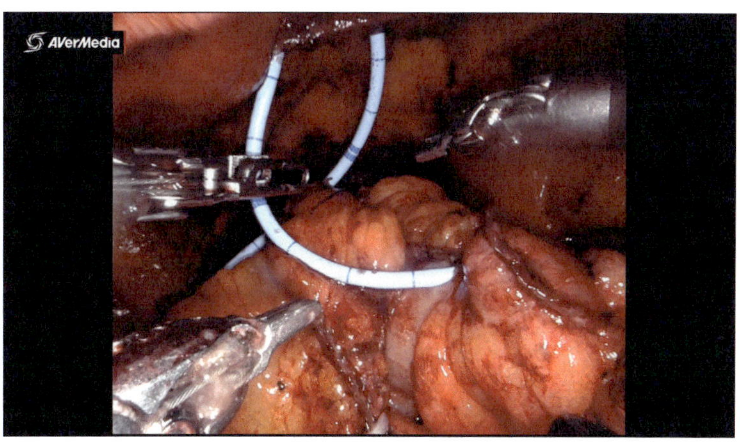

Figure 7.
Final two chimney neobladder formation with ureteral external stents.

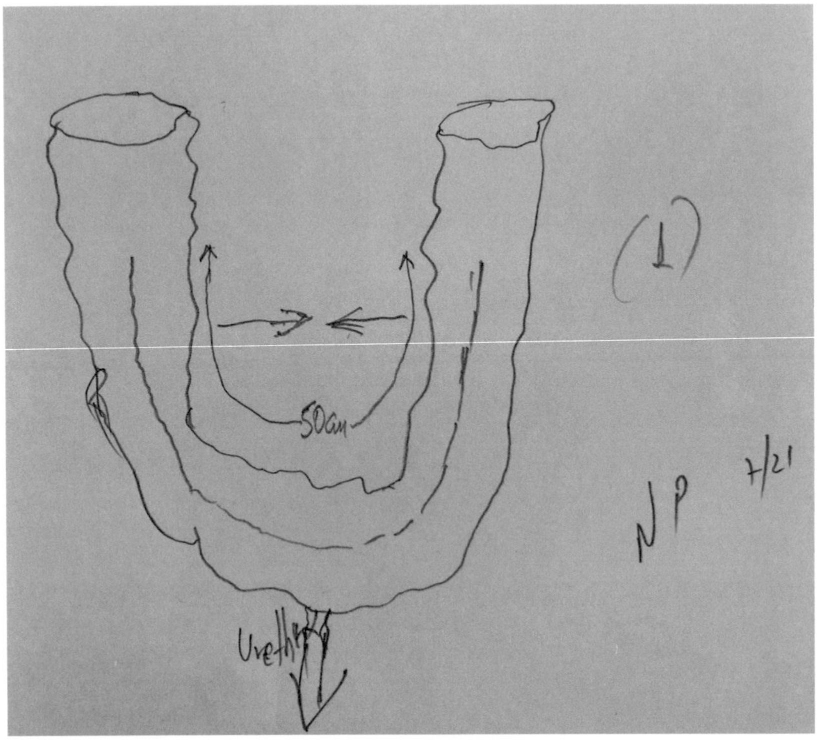

Figure 8.
Isolation of final ileal segment of 75 cm. A 12,5 cm part chimney is preserved in each side and the rest is detubularized.

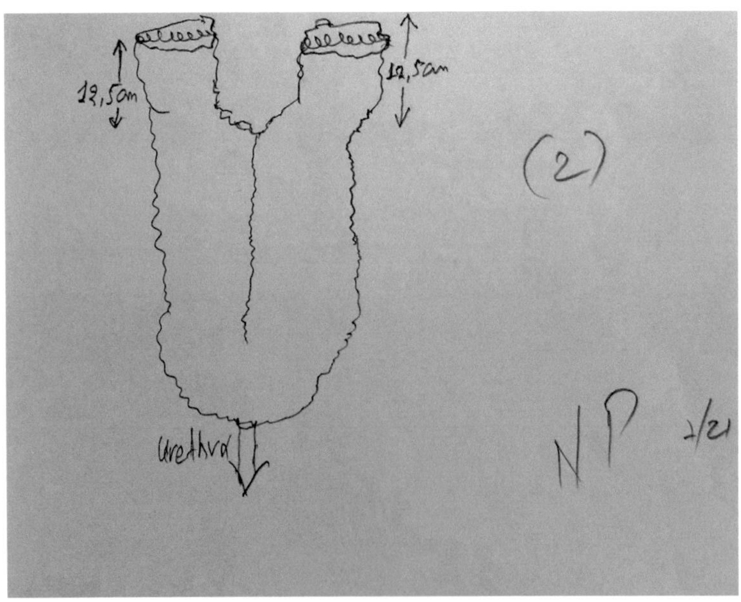

Figure 9.
The posterior part is anastomosed with 3.0 continuous sutures.

to access each anastomosis without damaging the other one [4]. We are using ureteral catheters on each side which are exteriorized to the skin and removed a week postoperatively. An ERAS protocol for quick recovery is a standard

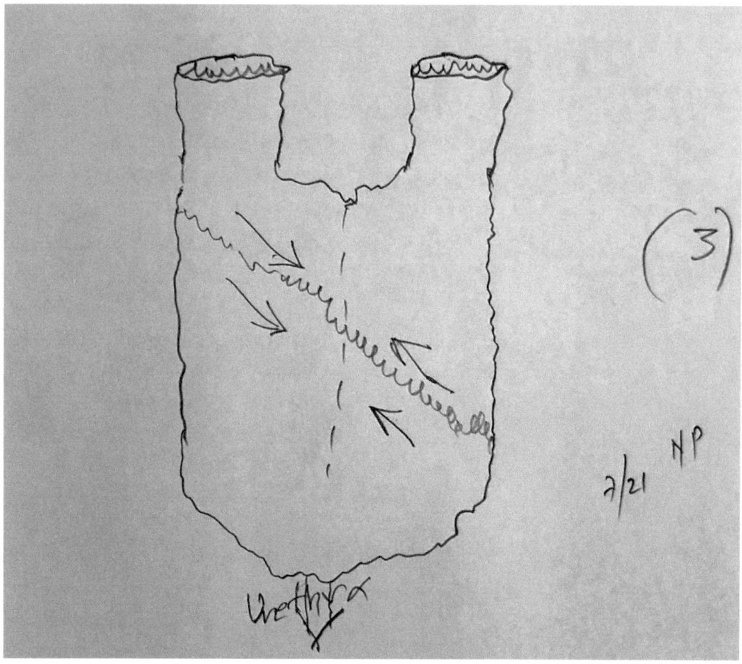

Figure 10.
The right upper part of the ileum is approached to the left lower part with continuous 3.0 sutures, creating a spheric neobladder.

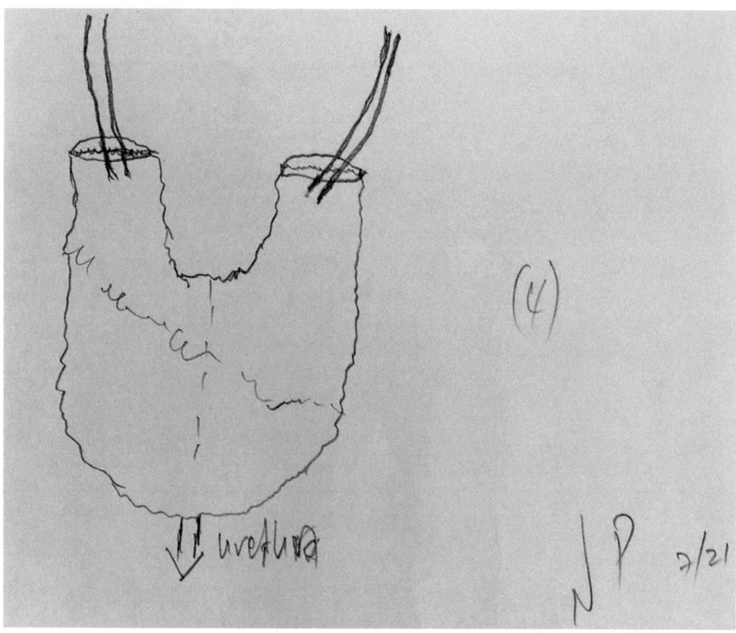

Figure 11.
The ureters are anastomosed with 4.0 sutures to each chimney seperately.

approach for the robotic cystectomy patients. In our last 5 patients we are performing a stentless watertight anastomosis with no stricture presence or hydronephrosis after a short of 18 months follow up time. These are very promising results.

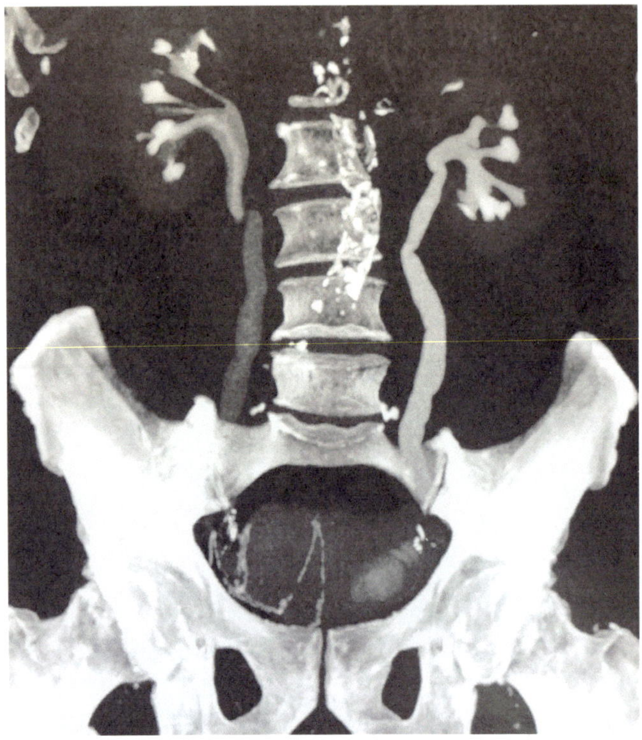

Figure 12.
CT urography follow up 2 years.

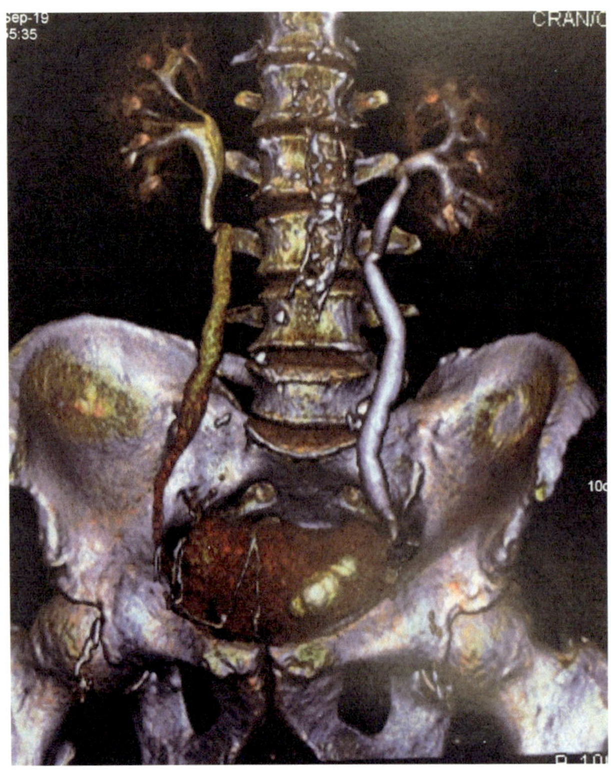

Figure 13.
CT urography follow up 10 years.

Urographic studies demonstrate no reflux or stricture in either of the implanted ureters (36 renal units in total), after 10 years of follow up (**Figures 12** and **13**) [5].

This modification of Studer neobladder with two chimneys is simple to handle, safe and free of ureteric stricture or reflux. With low stricture rates, this modified procedure of ureterointestinal anastomosis, is worthy of further promotion [6].

Author details

Panagiotis Pardalidis[1], Nikolaos Andriopoulos[2] and Nikolaos Pardalidis[2]*

1 Imperial School of Medicine, London, United Kingdom

2 Athens Medical Centre, Athens, Greece

*Address all correspondence to: npardali@otenet.gr

References

[1] Wein, A., Kavoussi, L., Partin, A., and Peters, C. Campbell-Walsh Urology. Eleventh Edition, Chapter 99. Philadelphia, PA: Elsevier. ISBN:978-1-4557-7567-5

[2] Dolezel, J. Ureterointestinal anastomosis in urinary diversion-current opinion. Rozhl Chir Spring 2017;96(4):146-150. PMID:28537409

[3] Schumacher, M. C., Jonsson, M. N., Hosseini, A., Nyberg, T., Poulakis, V., Pardalidis, N. P., John, H., and Wiklund, P. N. Surgery-related complications of robot-assisted radical cystectomy with intracorporeal urinary diversion. Urology 2011;77(4):871-876. DOI:10.1016/j.urology.2010.11.035

[4] Aguirre Benites, F., Duarte Ojeda, J. M., Pamplona Casamayor, M., Díaz González, R., and Leiva Galvis, O. Ileal neobladder with double chimney. Ureterointestinal anastomosis. Actas Urol Esp 2005;29(4):360-364. DOI:10.1016/s0210-4806(05)73256-3

[5] Abdelwahab, O., and Ahmed, M. M. M. Chimney modification technique for ureterointestinal anastomosis after radical cystectomy: Preliminary evaluation of short-term outcome and impact on quality of life. Curr Urol 2010;4:193-202.

[6] Ballouhey, Q., Thoulouzan, M., Lunardi, P., Bellec, L., Huyghe, E., Plante, P., de Petriconi, R., Soulié, M. Prospective study of the results of ureterointestinal anastomosis in 100 patients after the Hautmann ileal neobladder with double chimney. Prog Urol 2012;22(5):255-260. DOI:10.1016/j.purol.2011.11.005

Chapter 6

Advancements in Intravesical Chemotherapy in Non-Muscle Invasive Bladder Cancer

Ankur Mittal, Vikas Kumar Panwar and Gurpremjit Singh

Abstract

The treatment for non-muscle-invasive bladder cancer is transurethral resection of bladder cancer followed by intravesical chemotherapy or BCG. There have been various advancements in low risk, intermediate risk, high risk, and BCG failure cases of non-muscle invasive bladder cancer. There has been increased research on hyperthermia and intravesical chemotherapy, new agents like apaziquone, use of gemcitabine in low-risk cases, and combination chemotherapy in cases of BCG failure. Combining docetaxel and gemcitabine has taken a significant stage because of BCG shortage in some parts of the world. This chapter will discuss the latest advancements in intravesical chemotherapy in low, intermediate, and high-risk patients.

Keywords: Non-muscle invasive bladder cancer, Intravesical chemotherapy, Advancements in intravesical chemotherapy, Gemcitabine, Docetaxel, Nanoparticles, Mitomycin, Heated chemotherapy

1. Introduction

Bladder cancer accounts for 3% of the total cancers diagnosed in the world. It is more prevalent in developed countries. The most potent risk factor is tobacco smoking. Seventy-five percent of bladder cancer cases present with non-muscle invasive disease. The five-year survival statistics in the US are 69.5% for localized disease, 36.3% for regional disease, and only 4.6% for metastatic disease [1]. Almost three-fourths of high-risk non-muscle invasive bladder cancer will have a recurrence within ten years, 33% will progress to invasive disease [2].

Clinical guidelines suggest a risk-stratified approach post TURBT for intravesical therapy instillation. BCG has been the gold standard for intermediate and high-risk diseases. However, 61% of all patients recur within one year [3, 4]. In low-risk patients, a single post-operative instillation is adequate. This is based on a meta-analysis by Sylvester et al., which showed that patients receiving post-operative chemotherapy had a decrease in 39% of odds of recurrence with chemotherapy. They also showed that in patients with multiple tumors single instillation was not successful. Patients with a single tumor had a recurrence of 35.8% vs. a recurrence of 65.2% in patients with multiple tumors. No difference in different chemotherapeutic agents was found. The instillation is recommended to be given within 6 hours after TURBT, but in any case, within 24 hours if there is no deep resection [5].

The intermediate-risk group of patients is the largest group of non-muscle invasive bladder cancer patients. Intravesical instillations are recommended to decrease the risk of recurrence. The combined analysis from the European Organization for Research and Treatment of Cancer [EORTC] and Medical Research Council [MRC] randomized clinical trials included 2535 patients of primary or recurrent, stage TaT1 transitional cell carcinoma compared transurethral resection alone with and without adjuvant intravesical therapy. It showed a significant difference in terms of the duration of disease-free survival. No significant advantage in progression was seen. The median follow-up for survival was 7.8 years [6]. The guidelines recommend intravesical instillations of chemotherapeutic agents or BCG post TURBT in the intermediate-risk group [7, 8].

A second TURBT is mandatory within 2–6 weeks in the current guidelines in the high-risk group [7]. Guidelines recommend BCG intravesical therapy for high-risk patients. This is based on a meta-analysis by Sylvester et al., which included 24 trials with 4863 patients. The median follow-up was 2.5 years, and the maximum follow-up was of 15 years. In the BCG group, 260 out of 268 progressed [9.8%] while in the control group 304 out of 2205 progressed [13.8%]. There was a reduction of 27% in progression on BCG and the results were statistically significant. No significant benefit in disease-free survival was found [9]. No adjuvant chemotherapeutic regimens are included in the clinical guidelines as of now.

2. Advancements in low-risk disease

2.1 Gemcitabine

2.1.1 The rationale for using gemcitabine

Gemcitabine is 2′2’ – diflourodeoxycytidine and it has a broad spectrum of antitumor activity. It is phosphorylated and incorporated into DNA and RNA which results in apoptosis.

Many characteristics make gemcitabine a promising intravesical agent for bladder cancer. First, there has been a response rate of 27–38% during the systematic administration of gemcitabine against invasive bladder cancer. Second, the absorption of intravesical chemotherapeutic agents requires the size of the drug to be less than 300 Da. Gemcitabine has a molecular weight of 299 Da, which is lower than mitomycin and doxorubicin. It enables the drug to better penetrate the bladder mucosa and at the same time, the molecular weight is not too low so that systematic absorption of the drug occurs. The pKa of the drug is 3.6 and it results in a pH of 2.7–3.2 after reconstitution. Therefore, it results in low ionization of the drug at the acidic pH of the urine [10].

2.1.2 Studies for intravesical gemcitabine

Bohle et al. conducted a double-blind placebo-controlled randomized control trial in low and intermediate-risk patients for post-TURBT intravesical gemcitabine versus placebo in 355 patients in 24 urological centers. They used a single post-operative instillation of 2gm in 100 ml NS of gemcitabine with a 30–40 minutes retention time. The placebo used was 100 ml of normal saline. Both of these were followed by 20-hour bladder irrigation. The median follow-up was 24 months. Recurrence-free survival [12 months] was 77.7% in the gemcitabine group and 75.3% in the placebo group. There was no statistical significance between the two groups. The authors concluded that continuous irrigation and improved TURBT techniques might have led to high recurrence-free survival in both groups [11].

The SWOG SO337 randomized control trial was conducted at 23 US centers, and it assessed the effect of single post-operative instillation of intravesical gemcitabine versus saline in low-risk NMIBC cases. They used 2gm gemcitabine in 100 ml NS and 100 ml saline with a retention time of 1 hour in both groups. A total of 215 patients with low-risk NMIBC were randomized. The median follow-up was four years. In the gemcitabine group, 34 recurred out of 102, and in the saline group, 59 recurred out of 113 patients. There was a statistically significant difference between both groups [P = 0.001]. There were no grade 4 or 5 adverse events. The authors concluded that in low-risk non muscle-invasive bladder cancer patients, immediate intravesical instillation of gemcitabine significantly reduced the recurrence rate over a median of 4 years [12].

2.2 Apaziquone

Apaziquone is a mitomycin derivative and chemically 5-[aziridin-1-yl]-3-[hydroxymethyl]-2-[[1E]-3-hydroxyprop-1-enyl]-1-methyl-1H-indole-4,7-dione. It has a molecular weight of 288.30 Da. The drug product is called EOquin, and it has a storage temperature of 2–8 degrees Celsius. Before intravesical instillation, the EOquin vial is reconstituted with 20 ml of Diluent [a propylene glycol solution for intravesical instillation] to yield 0.2 mg/ml of apaziquone. This solution is further diluted with 20 ml of sterile water for injection, USP, resulting in 40 ml of the instillation solution containing 0.1 mg/ml of apaziquone [13].

It is the most potent intravesical agent in vitro. It is a prodrug and enzymatically activated by DT diaphorase [DTD] to generate cytotoxic species [13].

Karsh et al. reported two phases 2 multinational, double-blind placebo-controlled trials in patients with Ta, G1-G2 NMIBC to evaluate the efficacy of single instillation of apaziquone post TURBT. These two trials [SPI -611 and SPI 612] were conducted between April 2007 to January 2012. A single intravesical instillation of apaziquone [4 mg/40 mL] or placebo was administered within 6 hours post-TURBT. The primary endpoint was a 2-year recurrence-free rate, and the secondary endpoint was time to recurrence. A total of 1614 patients were enrolled.

Individually the two studies did not meet any statistical significance for a 2-year recurrence-free rate [38.0% vs. 44.6%, 39.7% vs. 46.3%]. When the pooled analysis was presented, it showed a 6.7% reduction in the 2-year recurrence-free rate. [OR – 0.76, P – 0.0218]. In both the studies, time to recurrence showed improvement, which was statistically significant in the SPI-611 study. Pooled data for time to recurrence also showed a significant improvement of time-to-recurrence [hazard ratio [HR] 0.79; P5.0096]. Apaziquone is rapidly metabolized in the blood. Therefore, a post hoc analysis was conducted by the time window of drug instillation post TURBT. Patients who had drugs instilled in the time window 60 ± 30 minutes post-TURBT demonstrated 20.3% and 20.8% reduction in 2- in the two studies, respectively.

These studies reported the safety of this drug for intravesical instillation, but further studies are required for determining the efficacy of this drug [14].

3. Advancements in intermediate and high-risk disease

3.1 Heated intravesical chemotherapy

Hyperthermia is the application of mild heat [40–44-degree Celsius]. Thermal ablation is having a higher temperature range of 60^0 to 90^0 Celsius. Hyperthermia helps in triggering the immune anti-cancer response. It also helps to improve drug delivery and is itself also directly cytotoxic to the cancer cells [15, 16].

The warm temperature results in local vasodilation and causes the leaky tumor vasculature to become leakier, resulting in improved drug delivery to the tumor cells. This is called the enhanced permeability and retention effect [17]. Hyperthermia can be provided by external devices and internal devices. Internal devices are most commonly used. **Table 1** describes the various devices which are used.

Heated intravesical chemotherapy has been used in neoadjuvant and adjuvant settings.

3.1.1 Neoadjuvant setting

Sousa et al., conducted a pilot clinical trial in 15 patients with intermediate and high-risk non-muscle-invasive bladder cancer patients. HIVEC consisting of eight weekly instillations of intravesical mitomycin C [80 mg in 50 mL] delivered with the novel Combat BRS® system at a temperature of 43°C for 60 min. A total of 119 treatments sessions were given. During TURBT it was found that 8 patients [53%] had a complete response and 7 [47%] had a partial response. The median follow-up was 29 months and the 3-year recurrence rate was 15%. No grade 3 toxicity was observed [18].

3.1.2 Adjuvant setting

Arends et al. conducted a phase III open-label, randomized control trial among 190 intermediate and high-risk non-muscle-invasive bladder cancer patients. 1-yr hyperthermia with mitomycin C [20 mg/50 mL] for 2, 30-minute sessions for six weeks, and maintenance course three cycles] were administered. The primary end-point was 24-month recurrence-free survival. The 24 months recurrence-free survival was 78.1% in the hyperthermia group and 64.8% in the BCG group [P = 0.08]. There was less than a 2% progression rate in both groups. No new adverse events were noted. In the per-protocol analysis, the 24 months recurrence-free survival was 81.8% in the hyperthermia group and 64.8% in the BCG group [P = 0.02]. The authors concluded that hyperthermia with Mitomycin C is safe and has a higher 2-year recurrence-free survival [21].

3.2 Ongoing trial for primary chemoablation

An ongoing phase 2 study of UGN-102 for low-grade intermediate risk non-muscle invasive bladder cancer [OPTIMA II] has enrolled 63 participants. They used 75 mg Mitomycin C [mitomycin C] in 56 mL admixture [1.33 mg mitomycin C per 1 mL of admixture], and six intravesical instillations were given weekly. The

Device	Mechanism of action
Combat bladder recirculating system [BRS] [Inno Medicus, Cham, Switzerland] [18]	Externally heat fluid and the circulate it to the bladder via a 3-way irrigating Foley catheter.
Unithermia [El Medical, Hod-Hasharon, Israel] [19]	Externally heat fluid and the circulate it to the bladder via a 3-way irrigating Foley catheter.
Synergo [Tigard, OR] [20]	Intravesical bladder heating system also uses recirculating bladder irrigation, but instead of a heat exchanger, it uses a microwave radiofrequency emitting intravesical catheter to heat the bladder.

Table 1.
The internal devices used for hyperthermia.

primary objective was the complete response rate three months after treatment. The trial completion date was December 2020, and results are awaited [22].

3.3 Gemcitabine docetaxel combination in BCG naive patients

Thomas et al. published an abstract of retrospective data for patients receiving sequential gemcitabine and docetaxel. The patients had not received any other intravesical therapy before. They were treated with six weekly instillations of gemcitabine [1 gram of gemcitabine in 50 ml of sterile water] followed immediately by docetaxel [37.5 mg of docetaxel in 50 mL of saline]. Maintenance therapy was then given for two years in patients without recurrence. The total number of patients identified was 30, and the median follow-up was 18 months. The indications of using this combination therapy were advanced age, immunosuppression, and BCG shortage. Treatment success was 96% at three months, 89% at one year, and 89% at two years. Treatment was well tolerated [23].

3.4 Ongoing trial for BCG naïve NMIBC: GEMDOCE trial

A phase II, two-stage, open-label trial for studying the safety and efficacy of gemcitabine docetaxel combination has started recruitment from Jul 29, 2020. The estimated enrolment is 26 patients, and the estimated completion is June 2024. The drug combination and dosing being used is 1 g gemcitabine in 50 ml sterile water; instilled once weekly for six weeks and then once monthly for ≤21 months and 37.5 mg docetaxel in 50 ml normal saline solution [NSS]; instilled once weekly for six weeks and then once monthly for ≤21 months. The primary objective is three months' complete response rate as assessed by cystoscopy and cytology. [ClinicalTrials.gov Identifier: NCT04386746] [24].

4. Advancements in BCG failure cases

4.1 Hyperthermia in BCG unresponsive cases

The HYMN trial was an open-label, two-arm, phase III randomized control trial in which 104 patients with BCG unresponsive non-muscle invasive bladder cancer were randomized to hyperthermia plus mitomycin or a second course of BCG. In the hyperthermia arm Synergo SB-TS 101 System was used and two 30 min cycles, each with 20 mg mitomycin at 42^0 +/− 2^0. Patients allocated to the BCG arm received six consecutive weekly BCG instillations [in 50 ml normal saline] followed by maintenance therapy [three consecutive weekly instillations at 3, 6, 12, 18, and 24 months]. Primary outcomes were disease-free survival [DFS] and three months complete response for CIS patients at randomization. The median follow-up was 35 months. No statistically significant difference was observed between the two arms. The hyperthermia arm had 35% DFS, and the BCG arm had 41% DFS. [HR 1.33, 95% confidence.

interval [CI] 0.84–2.10], p = 0.23; adjusted p = 0.49]. There was a nonsignificant higher DFS favoring hyperthermia group than BCG group in non-CIS patients at baseline [HR 0.50, 95% CI 0.22–1.17, p = 0.11] [25].

The most adverse events in this study were grades 1–2. There was two grade 4 toxicities in the BCG arm due to arthritis, and the other BCG-related sepsis resulted in death. No difference in health-related quality of life [HRQoL] was observed between the two treatment arms, although hyperthermia group patients reported their HRQoL higher than BCG group patients at 3,6 and 9 months [25].

4.2 Docetaxel

Docetaxel as a sole agent was studied in a phase I/II trial in 54 BCG refractory NMIBC between 2003 and 2012. A dose-escalation scheme was used in the first 18 patients treated with doses ranging from 5 to 75 mg for a final concentration of 0.125 to 0.75 mg/ml for administration. All subsequent patients received the maximum dose of 75 mg/100 ml of normal saline. All patients received six weekly instillations of intravesical docetaxel. After the phase I trial, those with a complete response to induction treatment were offered single dose monthly maintenance treatments for a total of up to 12 months of docetaxel therapy. The Median follow-up was 39.1 months. A complete initial response was seen in 32 patients [59%]. One year and the three-year recurrence-free rate was 40% and 25%, respectively. The authors concluded that intravesical docetaxel appears to be an efficacious agent, but large trials are needed to fully characterize this agent's benefits [26].

4.3 Gemcitabine and associated combinations

4.3.1 Gemcitabine as a sole agent

Gemcitabine has been studied in BCG refractory cases in two trials. Lorenzo et al. conducted a multi-center prospective randomized phase 2 trial in which 80 patients failing one course of BCG were randomly allocated to Gemcitabine arm and 2nd course of BCG arm. Kaplan Meier statistics of 2-year recurrence-free survival showed a significant difference between the gemcitabine and BCG group [19% and 3%, respectively, $P < 0.008$]. Seven of 21 [33%] patients in gemcitabine group and 13 of 35 [37.5%] patients in group had disease progression and underwent radical cystectomy [$P = .12$]. No significant safety concern was seen in both groups. The authors concluded that gemcitabine might be considered a second-line treatment after BCG failure in a high-risk non-muscle-invasive group [27].

Addeo et al. conducted a phase III randomized control trial in 120 high-risk NMIBC patients previously treated with BCG from march 2003 to November 2005. They received 40 mg of mitomycin C or 2000 mg of gemcitabine diluted in 50 mL of normal saline. The median follow-up was 36 months. In the gemcitabine arm, 39 of 54 patients remained free of recurrence versus 33 of 55 in the mitomycin C arm. Progression was seen in 10 patients in the mitomycin C arm and 6 in the gemcitabine arm. The incidence of chemical cystitis in the mitomycin C arm was statistically higher than in the gemcitabine arm [$P = .012$] [28].

These studies show that gemcitabine alone or combined can be considered in BCG refractory high-grade disease if cystectomy is contraindicated or refused [29].

4.3.2 Gemcitabine plus cabazitaxel plus cisplatin

A phase I trial studied the effect of this combination therapy. The trial was a dose-escalation, drug escalation study in patients of high-risk BCG failure NMIBC. A total of 18 patients were included, and the median follow-up was 27.8 months. The schedule used was

- 6-wk induction regimen of sequentially administered cabazitaxel, gemcitabine, and cisplatin

- Responders continued with maintenance cabazitaxel and gemcitabine monthly for the first year and bimonthly for the second year.

The dosing used in this study was:

1. Gemcitabine- 2 g/100 ml, Cabazitaxel – 5 mg/100 ml, Cis – 66 mg/100 ml

2. Gemcitabine- 2 g/100 ml, Cabazitaxel – 5 mg/100 ml, Cis – 80 mg/100 ml

3. Gemcitabine- 2 g/100 ml, Cabazitaxel – 5 mg/100 ml, Cis – 100 mg/100 ml

A complete response rate of 94% was observed, and a DFS of 78% was observed at 9.5 months. No Dose-limiting toxicity till the last follow-up. Further studies need to be done to evaluate the efficacy of this combination.

4.3.3 Gemcitabine plus mitomycin

This combination was first used in 2006, and it showed promising results in BCG failure patients. There were 20 months of median disease-free survival in the study by Maymi et al. [30].

In a retrospective study conducted by Cockerill et al., 27 patients with BCG failure were identified and had received gemcitabine plus mitomycin combination therapy. With a median follow-up of 22.1 months, ten patients had no recurrence. The authors concluded that this combination could offer durable recurrence-free survival to patients with recurrent NMIBC who are not candidates for, or refuse, cystectomy [31].

Similarly, Lightfoot et al. showed in a retrospective review of 47 patients who received six weekly treatments with sequential intravesical gemcitabine [1 g] and MMC [40 mg] chemotherapy for NMIBC. The median time for follow-up was 26 months. Fourteen of 47 patients [30%] remained free of recurrence. These studies show that gemcitabine plus mitomycin combination can be helpful in high-risk BCG failure NMIBC cases.

4.3.3.1 Administration of gemcitabine plus mitomycin combination

Patients should be pre-treated with an oral urinary alkalization agent [such as sodium bicarbonate the night before and the morning of installation]. Gemcitabine does not directly irritate the bladder, but its solution is very acidic [pH - 2.6], whereby Mitomycin C is inactivated under acidic conditions, and it irritates the bladder.

Patients receive six weekly intravesical installations for induction, which includes administration of the following:

1. 1 g Gemcitabine is diluted in 50 mL normal saline [Dwell time: 90 minutes]

2. The bladder is drained without rinsing

3. Instill 40 mg Mitomycin is diluted in 20 mL sterile saline [Dwell time 90 minutes]

Monthly maintenance administrations are generally given for 1 to 2 years or until recurrence [31, 32].

4.3.4 Gemcitabine plus docetaxel

Docetaxel inhibits mitosis and cell division by inhibiting the microtubular assembly [33]. Preclinical studies have shown that gemcitabine acts as an exfoliant for urothelial cells. This increases the penetration of docetaxel and therefore has enhanced efficacy [34].

Retrospective studies have shown that this combination is a promising intravesical combination in BCG failure cases. Milbar et al. showed in a retrospective analysis of 33 BCG unresponsive patients that 1-year recurrence-free survival [RFS] is 49% and 34% in 2 years [35]. Steinberg et al., in another retrospective analysis of 45 patients, showed treatment success of 66% at first surveillance, 54% at one year, and 34% at two years [36].

Steinberg et al. presented the preliminary results from a multi-institutional retrospective study of 276 BCG failure patients. The median follow-up was 22.9 months. Recurrence-free survival after 1 and 2 years was 60% and 46%, respectively. High-grade recurrence-free survival rates were 65% and 52%, respectively [37].

4.3.4.1 Administration of gemcitabine and docetaxel

The patient should be pre-treated with an oral alkalinizer. Pre-treatment with ondansetron helps to control gemcitabine-induced vomiting. Six intravesical instillations are given for induction as follows:

- 1 gm gemcitabine in 50 ml NS with a dwell time of 90 minutes.
- The bladder is drained without rinsing.
- 40 mg of docetaxel is diluted in 50 ml NS and given intravesical with a dwell time of 90–120 minutes.

Monthly maintenance is given 1–2 years [36, 37].

5. Nanoparticles

One nanometer is the scale at which many of the biological molecules operate inside the living cells. Nanoparticles accumulate in tumor tissues. This occurs via the enhanced permeability and retention [EPR] effect because the tumor tissues have a more permeable vascular supply, and this allows the nanoparticles to enter the cell. Nanoparticles can be used for the encapsulation of poorly soluble drugs [38].

Abraxane - nanoparticle albumin-bound version of paclitaxel. Nanoparticle albumin bound-paclitaxel has five times higher solubility as compared to docetaxel. Mckiernan et al. have studied this nanoparticle albumin-bound paclitaxel in 28 patients in a phase I single-center trial. Complete response was seen in 10 patients. The Median follow-up was 21 months. There was no progression in 19 out of28 patients. Their adverse events were limited to grades 1 and 2. The authors concluded that intravesical nab-paclitaxel had a 35.7% response rate in patients with NMIBC and BCG failure.

6. Future directions

After many years of stagnation, multiple new therapies are being investigated as potential intravesical agents for NMIBC. Strict criteria to define the disease have encouraged trials for patients with NMIBC. Most active trials focus on high-risk NMIBC in BCG naïve and BCG failure settings [39]. Multiple combination therapies continue to emerge. **Table 2** shows the various ongoing trials based on intravesical chemotherapy.

Trial	Phase	Drug used	Trial number
Neoadjuvant Short-term Intensive Chemoresection Versus Standard Adjuvant Intravesical Instillations in NMIBC	III	Mitomycin C	NCT03348969
CALIBER - A Phase II Randomized Feasibility Study of Chemoresection and Surgical Management in Low Risk Non-Muscle Invasive Bladder Cancer	I	Mitomycin C	NCT02070120
A Randomized, Single-Dose, Double-Blind, Placebo-Controlled Phase 3 Study of Qapzola™ [Apaziquone] as a Chemotherapy Adjuvant to Transurethral Resection of Bladder Tumors in Patients with Low- To-Intermediate-Risk NMIBC [CONQUER]	III	Apaziquone	NCT03224182 CONQUER
Evaluation of Immediate Preoperative Instillation [IPOI] of Mitomycin C Compared to Early Post-operative Instillation [IPOP] in Non-muscle Invasive Bladder Cancer	III	Mitomycin C	NCT02075060
A Phase 1/2a Pilot Study of Intravesical TSD-001 for Treatment of Low-Grade, Stage Ta, Non-Muscle Invasive Bladder Cancer	I	TSD-001	NCT03081858
A Prospective, Open-label Randomized Clinical Trial of a Single Bladder Instillation of Mitomycin C vs. Gemcitabine vs. No Additional Treatment Immediately After Transurethral Resection of Bladder Tumor [TURBT]	III	Mitomycin C Gemcitabine	NCT02695771
The Effectiveness and Safety of Neoadjuvant Intravesical Mitomycin-C Instillation in Non-muscle Invasive Bladder Cancer Patients: Prospective, Randomized, Phase II Study	III	Mitomycin C	NCT03058757
Open clinical trial to evaluate the efficacy of intravesical instillation of hyaluronate added to early instillation of mitomycin vs. early instillation of mitomycin in patients suffering from low risk not muscle-infiltrating bladder cancer	I	Hyaluronate Chondroitin sulfate	EUCTR2016–003813-92
A Phase 1b, Multicenter, Open Label Study Evaluating Safety, Tolerability and Preliminary Efficacy of GemRIS 225 mg in Subjects with Non-Muscle-Invasive Urothelial Carcinoma of the Bladder	III	Gemcitabine	NCT02720367
Randomized prospective clinical trial to evaluate the rate of early recurrence in non-muscle invasive bladder cancer between the chemohyperthermia [QH] with mitomycin-C prior to transurethral resection of bladder in ambulatory surgery program and post resection treatment with mitomycin C in normothermia.	III	Mitomycin C	EUCTR2015–005151-27
HIVEC HR: Use of chemohyperthermia with intravesical mitomycin [HIVEC] for the treatment of patients with NMIBC	I	Mitomycin C BCG	EUCTR2016–001186-85
HIVEC [Hyperthermic IntraVesical Chemotherapy] for Patients with Intermediate Risk NMIBC Compared with Standard Intravesical Instillation Of Chemotherapy As Adjuvant Treatment. A Comparative, Prospective, Randomized Study.	III	Mitomycin C	EUCTR2013–002628-18

Trial	Phase	Drug used	Trial number
A Phase 3 Study to Evaluate the Efficacy and Safety of Intravesical Nanoxel®M [Docetaxel-PM] In Bacillius Calmette-Guerin Refractory Non-Muscle Invasive Bladder Cancer	III	Docetaxel-PM Mitomycin-C	NCT02982395
A Phase I Trial for the Use of Intravesical Cabazitaxel, Gemcitabine, and Cisplatin [CGC] in the Treatment of BCG-Refractory Non-muscle Invasive Urothelial Carcinoma of the Bladder	I	Cabazitaxe Gemcitabine Cisplatin	NCT02202772
A Multi-center, Single-Arm Study Evaluating the Efficacy of Synergo® Radiofrequency-Induced Thermochemotherapy Effect [RITE] With Mitomycin C [Synergo® RITE + MMC] in CIS Non-Muscle Invasive Bladder Cancer [NMIBC] Bacillus Calmette-Guérin [BCG]-Unresponsive Patients with or without Papillary NMIBC	III	Synergo RITE + MMC	NCT03335059

Table 2.
The ongoing clinical trials based on intravesical chemotherapeutic agents.

Food and drug administration gave guidelines on designing trials in NMIBC as follows: [40].

- High-risk NMIBC

  1. Trials can include a mix of high risk and CIS cases
  2. Time to an event is the preferred endpoint
  3. Placebo-controlled trials of BCG are not helpful.
  4. The duration of follow-up should be at least 18–24 months.

- High-risk BCG refractory

  1. No standard of care in this group.
  2. Single-arm trials can be used if they provide robust results
  3. Patients having BCG refractory CIS should have a complete response rate of 40–50% at six months and at least 30% response rate at 18–24 months.

- Placebo trials

  These can be used in low-risk patients.

- Perioperative intravesical instillation agents

  1. Time to event analysis should be used
  2. Follow-up of at least two years
  3. The clinically meaningful result is defined as a 15% event rate reduction or a hazard ratio of 0.7.

7. Conclusion

The **Table 3** and **Figure 1** summarizes the various advancements in intravesical chemotherapy in NMIBC and **Figure 1** also gives the intravesical chemotherapy of choice in various risk categories.

Risk	Advancement
Low risk	• Gemcitabine can also be used as a 1st line agent for single instillation post TURBT
Intermediate and high-risk BCG naive	• Single agent - HIVEC + MMC show favorable response. • Combination – Gemcitabine + Docetaxel combination is under research
BCG failure	• Gemcitabine alone or in combination can be if cystectomy is contraindicated or refused.

Table 3.
Summary of the various advancements in intravesical chemotherapy in NMIBC.

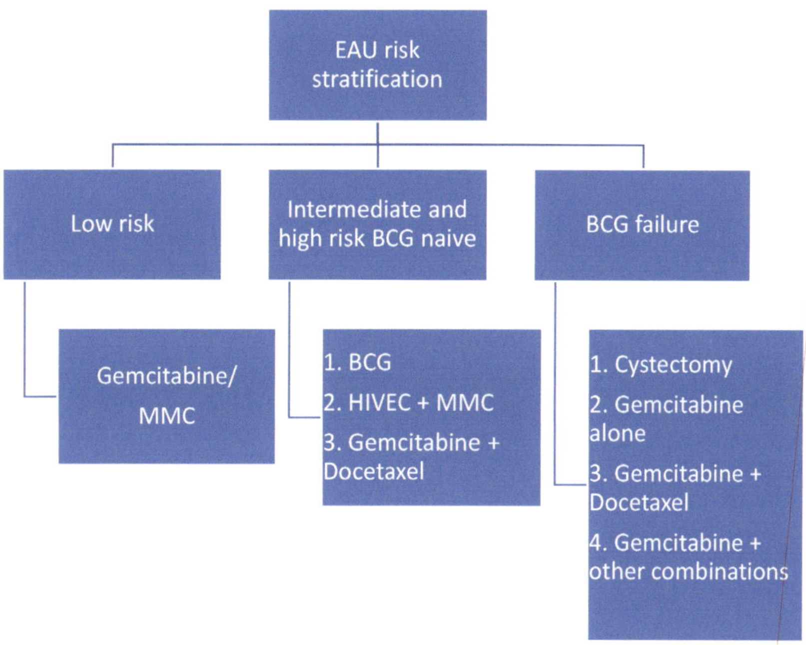

Figure 1.
EAU risk stratification based intravesical chemotherapy of choice in various risk categories.

Conflict of interest

The authors declare no conflict of interest.

Appendices and nomenclature

European association of urology 2021 non-muscle invasive bladder cancer risk stratification:

Risk group stratification and Characteristics

1. **Low-risk tumors** - Primary, solitary, TaG1 [PUNLMP, LG*], < 3 cm, no CIS.

2. **Intermediate-risk tumors** - All tumors not defined in the two adjacent categories

3. **High-risk tumors** - Any of the following:

    - T1 tumor

    - G3 [HG**] tumor

    - carcinoma *in situ* [CIS]

    - Multiple, recurrent and large [> 3 cm] TaG1G2/LG tumors [all features must be present]

Author details

Ankur Mittal, Vikas Kumar Panwar and Gurpremjit Singh*
All India Institute of Medical Sciences, Rishikesh, India

*Address all correspondence to: gurpremjita7@gmail.com

References

[1] Cumberbatch MGK, Jubber I, Black PC, Esperto F, Figueroa JD, Kamat AM, et al. Epidemiology of Bladder Cancer: A Systematic Review and Contemporary Update of Risk Factors in 2018. Eur Urol. 2018;74[6]:784-95.

[2] Chamie K, Litwin MS, Bassett JC, Daskivich TJ, Lai J, Hanley JM, et al. recurrence of high-risk bladder cancer: a population-based analysis. Cancer. 2013 Sep 1;119[17]:3219-27.

[3] Fernandez-Gomez J, Madero R, Solsona E, Unda M, Martinez-Piñeiro L, Gonzalez M, et al. Predicting non-muscle invasive bladder cancer recurrence and progression in patients treated with bacillus Calmette-Guerin: the CUETO scoring model. J Urol. 2009 Nov;182[5]:2195-203.

[4] Sylvester RJ, van der Meijden APM, Oosterlinck W, Witjes JA, Bouffioux C, Denis L, et al. Predicting recurrence and progression in individual patients with stage Ta T1 bladder cancer using EORTC risk tables: a combined analysis of 2596 patients from seven EORTC trials. Eur Urol. 2006 Mar;49[3]:466-465; discussion 475-477.

[5] Sylvester RJ, Oosterlinck W, van der Meijden APM. A single immediate post-operative instillation of chemotherapy decreases the risk of recurrence in patients with stage Ta T1 bladder cancer: a meta-analysis of published results of randomized clinical trials. J Urol. 2004 Jun;171[6 Pt 1]:2186-90, quiz 2435.

[6] Pawinski A, Sylvester R, Kurth KH, Bouffioux C, van der Meijden A, Parmar MK, et al. A combined analysis of European Organization for Research and Treatment of Cancer, and Medical Research Council randomized clinical trials for the prophylactic treatment of stage TaT1 bladder cancer. European Organization for Research and Treatment of Cancer Genitourinary Tract Cancer Cooperative Group and the Medical Research Council Working Party on Superficial Bladder Cancer. J Urol. 1996 Dec;156[6]:1934-40, discussion 1940-1941.

[7] EAU. EAU Guidelines: Non-muscle-invasive Bladder Cancer [Internet]. Uroweb. [cited 2021 Feb 28]. Available from: https://uroweb.org/guideline/non-muscle-invasive-bladder-cancer/

[8] AUA. Bladder Cancer: Non-Muscle Invasive Guideline - American Urological Association [Internet]. [cited 2021 Feb 28]. Available from: https://www.auanet.org/guidelines/bladder-cancer-non-muscle-invasive-guideline

[9] Sylvester RJ, van der MEIJDEN APM, Lamm DL. Intravesical bacillus Calmette-Guerin reduces the risk of progression in patients with superficial bladder cancer: a meta-analysis of the published results of randomized clinical trials. J Urol. 2002 Nov;168[5]:1964-70.

[10] Gontero P, Marini L, Frea B. Intravesical gemcitabine for superficial bladder cancer: rationale for a new treatment option. BJU Int. 2005; 96[7]:970-6.

[11] Böhle A, Leyh H, Frei C, Kühn M, Tschada R, Pottek T, et al. Single post-operative instillation of gemcitabine in patients with non-muscle-invasive transitional cell carcinoma of the bladder: a randomised, double-blind, placebo-controlled phase III multicentre study. Eur Urol. 2009 Sep;56[3]:495-503.

[12] Messing EM, Tangen CM, Lerner SP, Sahasrabudhe DM, Koppie TM, Wood DP, et al. Effect of Intravesical Instillation of Gemcitabine vs Saline Immediately Following Resection of

Suspected Low-Grade Non-Muscle-Invasive Bladder Cancer on Tumor Recurrence: SWOG S0337 Randomized Clinical Trial. JAMA. 2018 08;319[18]: 1880-8.

[13] Witjes JA, Kolli PS. Apaziquone for non-muscle invasive bladder cancer: a critical review. Expert Opin Investig Drugs. 2008 Jul;17[7]:1085-96.

[14] Karsh L, Shore N, Soloway M, Bhat G, Reddy G, Leu S-Y, et al. Double-Blind, Randomized, Placebo-controlled Studies Evaluating Apaziquone [E09, Qapzola™] Intravesical Instillation Post Transurethral Resection of Bladder Tumors for the Treatment of Low-risk Non-Muscle Invasive Bladder Cancer. Bladder Cancer Amst Neth. 2018 Jul 30;4[3]:293-301.

[15] Frey B, Weiss E-M, Rubner Y, Wunderlich R, Ott OJ, Sauer R, et al. Old and new facts about hyperthermia-induced modulations of the immune system. Int J Hyperth Off J Eur Soc Hyperthermic Oncol North Am Hyperth Group. 2012;28[6]:528-42.

[16] Hildebrandt B, Wust P, Ahlers O, Dieing A, Sreenivasa G, Kerner T, et al. The cellular and molecular basis of hyperthermia. Crit Rev Oncol Hematol. 2002 Jul;43[1]:33-56.

[17] Maeda H, Tsukigawa K, Fang J. A Retrospective 30 Years After Discovery of the Enhanced Permeability and Retention Effect of Solid Tumors: Next-Generation Chemotherapeutics and Photodynamic Therapy--Problems, Solutions, and Prospects. Microcirc N Y N 1994. 2016 Apr;23[3]:173-82.

[18] Sousa A, Piñeiro I, Rodríguez S, Aparici V, Monserrat V, Neira P, et al. Recirculant hyperthermic IntraVEsical chemotherapy [HIVEC] in intermediate-high-risk non-muscle-invasive bladder cancer. Int J Hyperth Off J Eur Soc Hyperthermic Oncol North Am Hyperth Group. 2016 Jun;32[4]:374-80.

[19] Soria F, Milla P, Fiorito C, Pisano F, Sogni F, Di Marco M, et al. Efficacy and safety of a new device for intravesical thermochemotherapy in non-grade 3 BCG recurrent NMIBC: a phase I-II study. World J Urol. 2016 Feb;34[2]: 189-95.

[20] Rigatti P, Lev A, Colombo R. Combined intravesical chemotherapy with mitomycin C and local bladder microwave-induced hyperthermia as a preoperative therapy for superficial bladder tumors. A preliminary clinical study. Eur Urol. 1991;20[3]:204-10.

[21] Arends TJH, Nativ O, Maffezzini M, de Cobelli O, Canepa G, Verweij F, et al. Results of a Randomised Controlled Trial Comparing Intravesical Chemohyperthermia with Mitomycin C Versus Bacillus Calmette-Guérin for Adjuvant Treatment of Patients with Intermediate- and High-risk Non-Muscle-invasive Bladder Cancer. Eur Urol. 2016 Jun;69[6]:1046-52.

[22] UroGen Pharma Ltd. A Phase 2b, Single-Arm, Multicenter Trial to Evaluate the Efficacy and Safety of UGN-102 as Primary Chemoablative Therapy in Patients With Low Grade [LG] Non-Muscle-Invasive Bladder Cancer [NMIBC] at Intermediate Risk of Recurrence [Internet]. clinicaltrials.gov; 2020 Dec [cited 2021 Feb 28]. Report No.: study/NCT03558503. Available from: https://clinicaltrials.gov/ct2/show/study/NCT03558503

[23] Thomas L, Steinberg R, Nepple KG, O'Donnell MA. Sequential intravesical gemcitabine and docetaxel in the treatment of BCG-naive patients with non-muscle invasive bladder cancer. J Clin Oncol. 2019 Feb 26;37[7_suppl]:469-469.

[24] Sidney Kimmel Comprehensive Cancer Center at Johns Hopkins. A

Phase II Trial for the Use of Intravesical Gemcitabine and Docetaxel [GEMDOCE] in the Treatment of BCG naïve Non-muscle Invasive Urothelial Carcinoma of the Bladder [Internet]. clinicaltrials.gov; 2020 Aug [cited 2021 Feb 28]. Report No.: NCT04386746. Available from: https://clinicaltrials.gov/ct2/show/NCT04386746

[25] Tan WS, Panchal A, Buckley L, Devall AJ, Loubière LS, Pope AM, et al. Radiofrequency-induced Thermo-chemotherapy Effect Versus a Second Course of Bacillus Calmette-Guérin or Institutional Standard in Patients with Recurrence of Non-muscle-invasive Bladder Cancer Following Induction or Maintenance Bacillus Calmette-Guérin Therapy [HYMN]: A Phase III, Open-label, Randomised Controlled Trial. Eur Urol. 2019 Jan;75[1]:63-71.

[26] Barlow LJ, McKiernan JM, Benson MC. Long-term survival outcomes with intravesical docetaxel for recurrent non-muscle invasive bladder cancer after previous bacillus Calmette-Guérin therapy. J Urol. 2013 Mar;189[3]:834-9.

[27] Di Lorenzo G, Perdonà S, Damiano R, Faiella A, Cantiello F, Pignata S, et al. Gemcitabine versus bacille Calmette-Guérin after initial bacille Calmette-Guérin failure in non-muscle-invasive bladder cancer: a multicenter prospective randomized trial. Cancer. 2010 Apr 15;116[8]:1893-900.

[28] Addeo R, Caraglia M, Bellini S, Abbruzzese A, Vincenzi B, Montella L, et al. Randomized phase III trial on gemcitabine versus mytomicin in recurrent superficial bladder cancer: evaluation of efficacy and tolerance. J Clin Oncol Off J Am Soc Clin Oncol. 2010 Feb 1;28[4]:543-8.

[29] Shelley MD, Jones G, Cleves A, Wilt TJ, Mason MD, Kynaston HG. Intravesical gemcitabine therapy for non-muscle invasive bladder cancer [NMIBC]: a systematic review. BJU Int. 2012 Feb;109[4]:496-505.

[30] Maymi JL, Saltsgaver N, O'Donnell MA. 840: Intravesical Sequential Gemcitabine-Mitomycin Chemotherapy as Salvage Treatment for Patients with Refractory Superficial Bladder Cancer. J Urol [Internet]. 2006 Apr [cited 2021 Mar 3]; Available from: https://www.auajournals.org/doi/abs/10.1016/S0022-5347%2818%2933076-3

[31] Cockerill PA, Knoedler JJ, Frank I, Tarrell R, Karnes RJ. Intravesical gemcitabine in combination with mitomycin C as salvage treatment in recurrent non-muscle-invasive bladder cancer. BJU Int. 2016 Mar;117[3]: 456-62.

[32] Aj L, Bn B, Hm R, Ba E, Br K, Ma O. Multi-institutional analysis of sequential intravesical gemcitabine and mitomycin C chemotherapy for non-muscle invasive bladder cancer [Internet]. Urologic oncology. 2014 [cited 2021 Mar 3]. Available from: https://pubmed.ncbi.nlm.nih.gov/23510863/

[33] Herbst RS, Khuri FR. Mode of action of docetaxel - a basis for combination with novel anti-cancer agents. Cancer Treat Rev. 2003 Oct;29[5]:407-15.

[34] Pandey R, Jackson JK, Liggins R, Mugabe C, Burt HM. Enhanced taxane uptake into bladder tissues following co-administration with either mitomycin C, doxorubicin or gemcitabine: association to exfoliation processes. BJU Int. 2018 Nov;122[5]: 898-908.

[35] Milbar N, Kates M, Chappidi MR, Pederzoli F, Yoshida T, Sankin A, et al. Oncological Outcomes of Sequential Intravesical Gemcitabine and Docetaxel in Patients with Non-Muscle Invasive

Bladder Cancer. Bladder Cancer Amst Neth. 3[4]:293-303.

[36] Steinberg RL, Thomas LJ, O'Donnell MA, Nepple KG. Sequential Intravesical Gemcitabine and Docetaxel for the Salvage Treatment of Non-Muscle Invasive Bladder Cancer. Bladder Cancer Amst Neth. 2015 Apr 30;1[1]:65-72.

[37] Steinberg Ryan L., Thomas Lewis J., Brooks Nathan, Mott Sarah L., Vitale Andrew, Crump Trafford, et al. Multi-Institution Evaluation of Sequential Gemcitabine and Docetaxel as Rescue Therapy for Nonmuscle Invasive Bladder Cancer. J Urol. 2020 May 1;203[5]:902-9.

[38] He M-H, Chen L, Zheng T, Tu Y, He Q, Fu H-L, et al. Potential Applications of Nanotechnology in Urological Cancer. Front Pharmacol [Internet]. 2018 [cited 2021 Mar 4];9. Available from: https://www.frontiersin.org/articles/10.3389/fphar.2018.00745/full

[39] Nykopp TK, Batista da Costa J, Mannas M, Black PC. Current Clinical Trials in Non-muscle Invasive Bladder Cancer. Curr Urol Rep. 2018 Oct 24;19[12]:101.

[40] Jarow JP, Lerner SP, Kluetz PG, Liu K, Sridhara R, Bajorin D, et al. Clinical Trial Design for the Development of New Therapies for Nonmuscle-invasive Bladder Cancer: Report of a Food and Drug Administration and American Urological Association Public Workshop. Urology. 2014 Feb 1;83[2]:262-5.